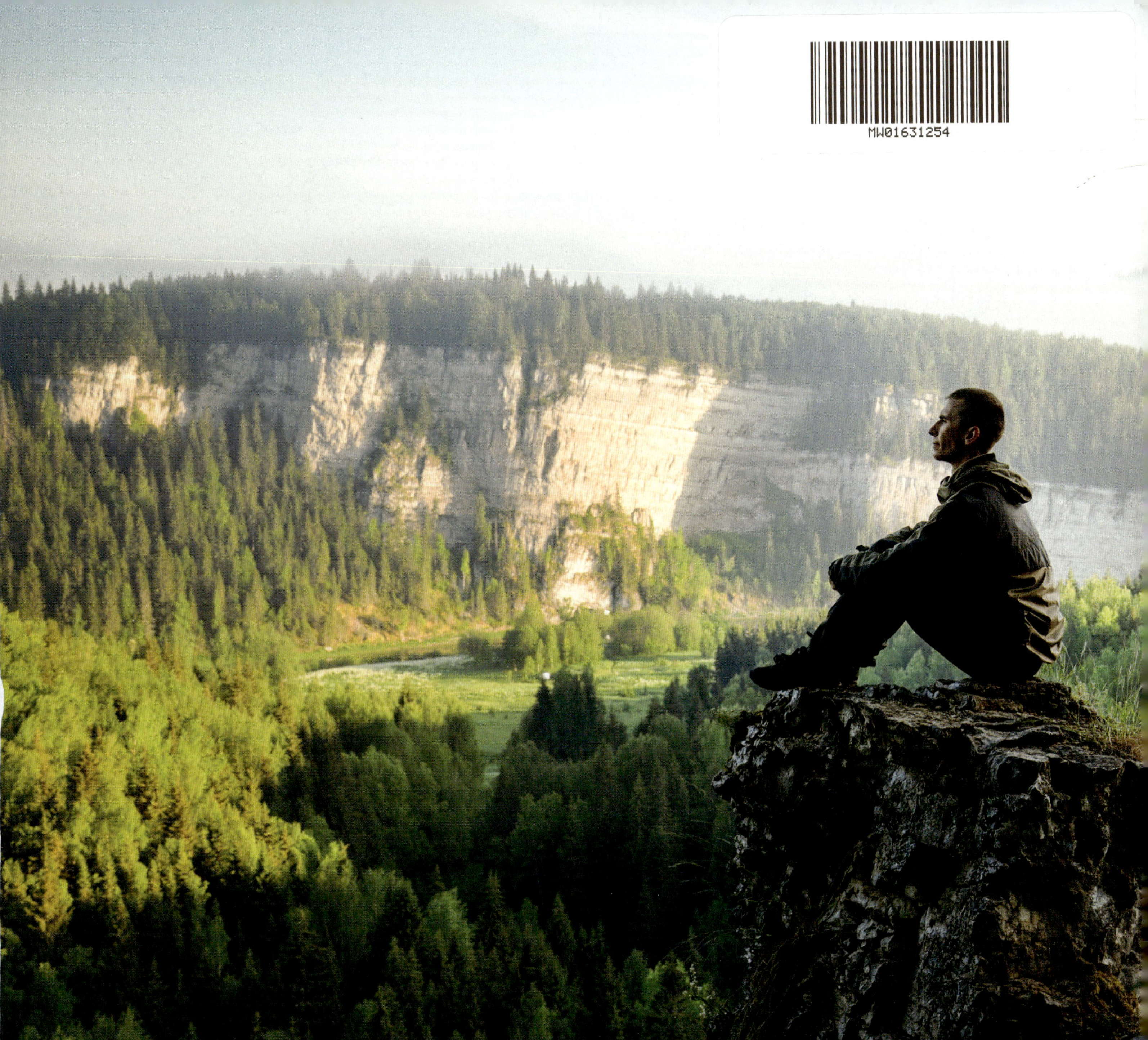

Maximizing Mindfulness

& Minimizing Stress

James E. Porter

Editorial Staff

Author: James E. Porter

Executive Editor: Aaron Hardy, MS

Designer: Integrated Health & Wellness

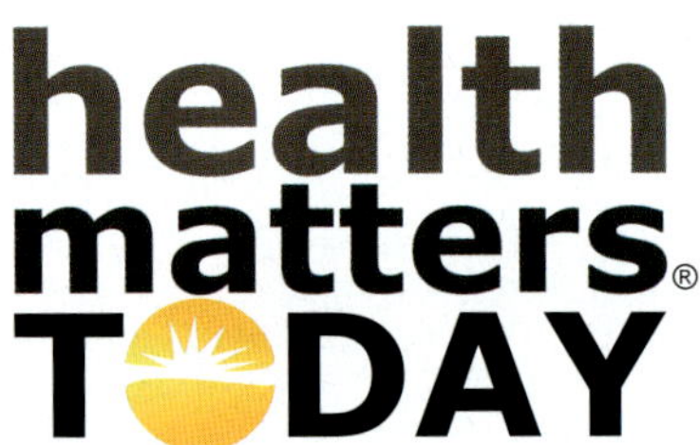

Integrated Health & Wellness
520 N. Main Street STE C422 | Heber City, UT 84032
Maximizing Human Capital | ihwsolutions.com

ISBN: 978-0-578-73532-0

Table of Contents

Chapter 1

What is Mindfulness?

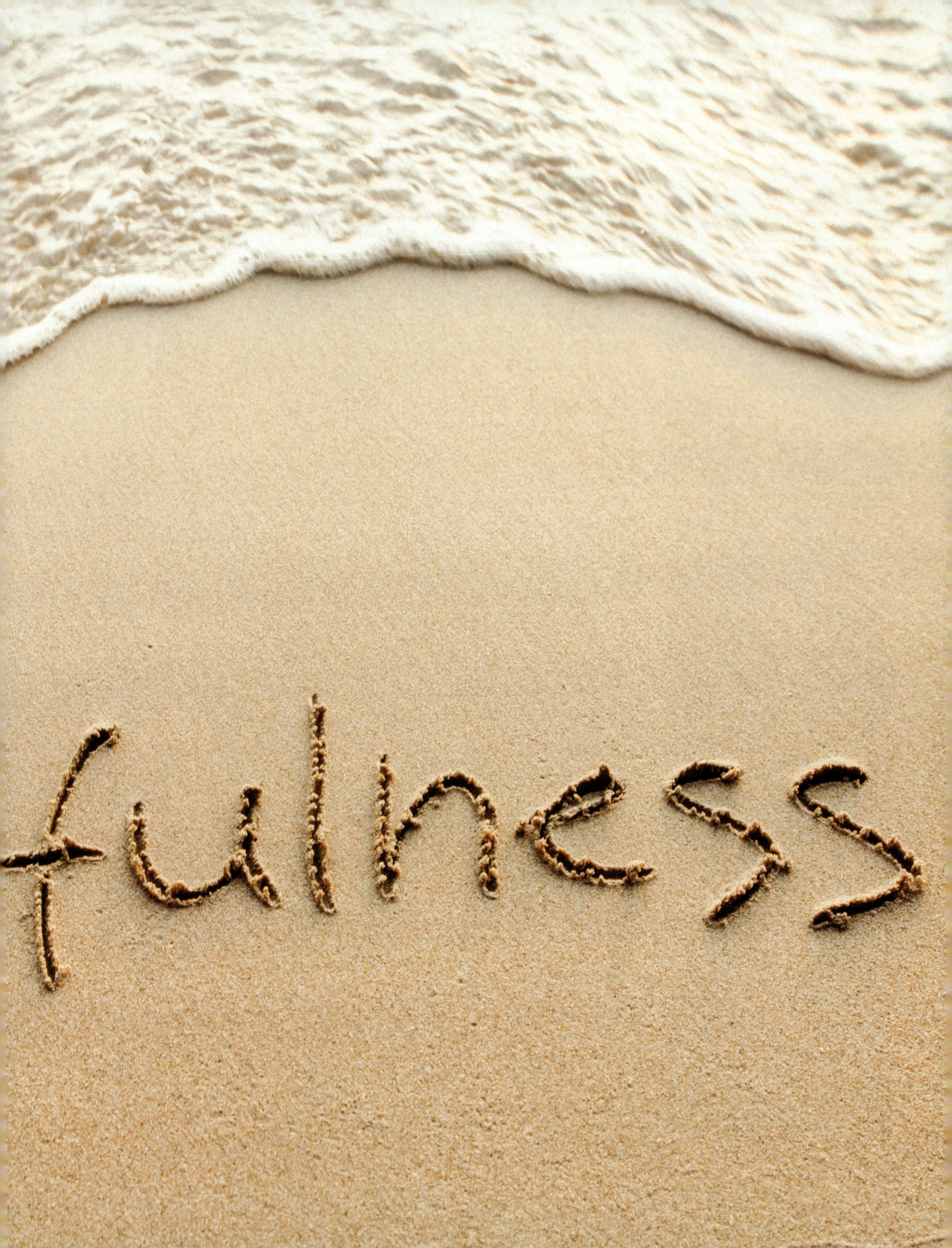
fulness

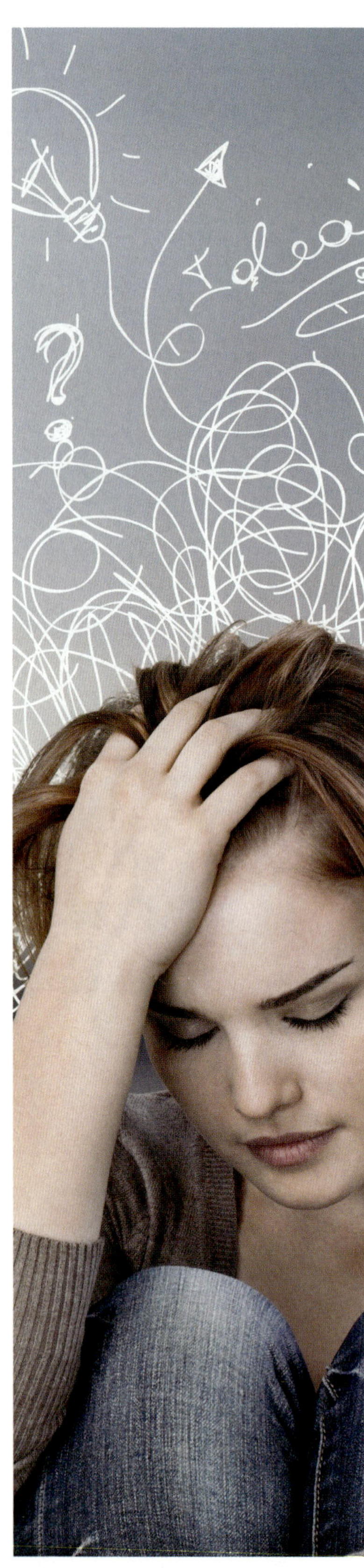

Chapter 1
What is Mindfulness?

Awareness doesn't get angry, anxious or depressed.

When I first encountered mindfulness, I completely rejected it. It was thirty years ago. I was reading an excerpt from a short book on mindfulness and the author was suggesting that I should wash my dishes mindfully: *Feel the hot water on the back of my hands, smell the dish detergent coming up to my nose, and listen to the sound of the scrub brush swirling around the pot.* I remember my reaction at the time was: *Isn't there anything better to think about?*

Like washing the dishes, there are so many different things we can do without thinking about it. From mowing the lawn to folding the laundry, our minds are often free to wander off and think about something other than what we are doing. This ability, to do one thing while thinking about another, is known as *automaticity*.

Automaticity helps us multi-task. We can walk through a crowded room while balancing two glasses of water on a tray on one hand while holding a pitcher full of lemonade in the other hand. We can talk on the phone while driving a car. We can take our eyes off the road and gaze at the scenery while riding a bike. These examples of multi-tasking may not seem so amazing but if you could remember back to when you were first learning how to walk, or ride a bike, or drive a car, you'd realize there was no automaticity then. These activities required your full attention. Now you do them on autopilot. You can do them *mindlessly*.

Whether it's ironing a shirt, making a bed, walking up a set of stairs, or putting away the dishes, we dedicate only a small portion of our attention (or possibly even NONE of it) to what we are *actually* doing.

Ever driven across town, zoned out for a few minutes, and ended up in parking lot across the street from where you had intended to go? Ever parked your car in the mall, only to realize two hours later, that you have NO IDEA where you parked it? Ever needed something from the kitchen but by the time you get there, you have *no idea* what you came in for? These are all examples of automaticity or *mindlessness*.

My favorite example of mindlessness is when I'm in the shower. I've been there for 10 or 15 minutes, my hair is wet, *but I have no idea whether I shampooed it or not.*

This happened to me just the other day. Instead of thinking about what I was doing, I was thinking about a dentist appointment I had the next day. Even though I was just getting my teeth cleaned, it suddenly occurred to me: *What if I have a cavity? What if I need a root canal?*

I haven't had a cavity in years, and I have NEVER had a root canal. But here I am. In the shower, IMAGINING what it MIGHT be like to get one.

The body believes what the mind conceives. What starts in the mind as a thought, often ends up in the body as a *very real* physical reaction. Have those kinds of negative thoughts often enough, and you can end up with a very real stress-related *dis-ease.*

So, I am standing in the shower, thinking about an event that probably will never happen, while stress chemicals like adrenalin and cortisol are being pumped into my bloodstream. As the result of these THOUGHTS, my blood pressure is starting to rise, my heart rate is starting to increase, and my muscles are becoming tense.[1]

At other times, *while in the shower,* my mind will go back in time and replay events that have already happened and can't be changed. At these times, I might be reviewing a negative interaction I've had with a coworker, my boss or my spouse. I will often replay these events over and over, making me angry and more upset.

Whether my mind wanders off into the future (where I get anxious) or back into the past, (where I get angry) either way, *it's not a good direction.* If I were to think about *what I was doing, while I was doing it*, not only would I be spared from both anxiety and anger, I would be experiencing something quite pleasurable instead. Now you can see the very practical value of *mindfulness.*

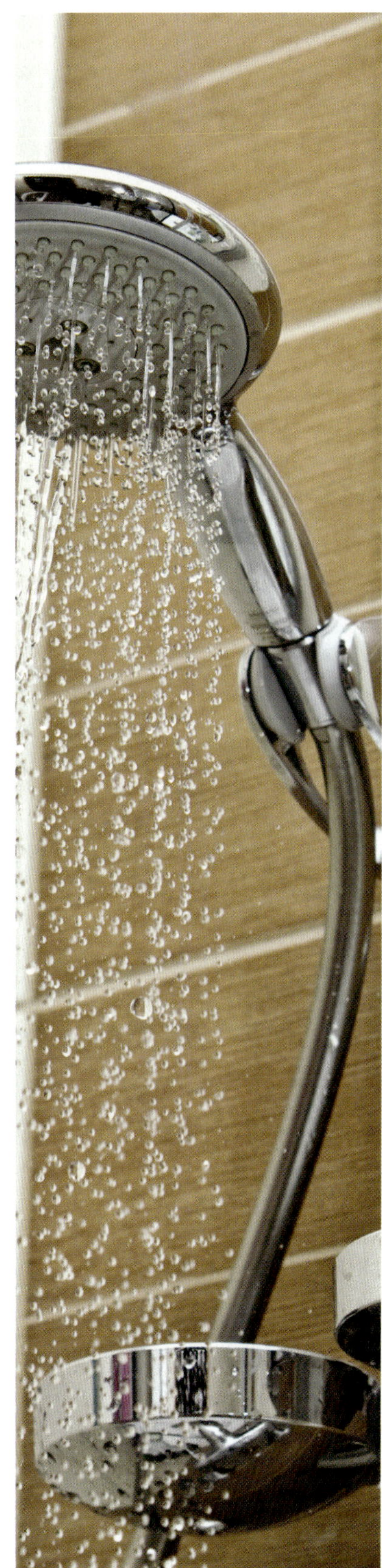

The shower (like a lot of other activities that we do daily) is a great place to BE mindful. It's like a spa in a box. Choose to think about what you are doing while you are doing it and not only are there medical benefits (which we discuss later), you will discover you have mentally created a safe haven from both anxiety and anger.

That's what I didn't understand when I first encountered mindfulness over twenty years ago. Sure, if while doing the dishes I was thinking about how wonderful my spouse was or how good my kids were, or if I was devising plans for a wonderful vacation, that would be a GREAT use of the mind's capacity to move both forward or backward in time.

But typically, the mind likes to dwell – in fact fixate or ruminate - on past or potential problems. However, *not in a way that might solve those problems.* Usually it's in a way that only makes them worse. (Which is why rumination is often linked to depression.)[2]

The opportunities to do things mindfully are everywhere you look. You can be more mindful when you eat, when you drive, and when you walk. When you live your life in this way, you will experience more joy, less stress, free yourself from distraction, get along better with your co-workers and be more productive. You'll even save time, have fewer errors and be able to concentrate better.

There are now thousands of "peer-reviewed" studies, published in medical and psychological journals that confirm the amazing benefits of mindfulness. Mindfulness practice has been proven to decrease tension, reduce stress and lower anxiety. It has been used to treat people with depression, eating disorders, addiction and even chronic pain. It's also been shown to improve immune system functioning, speed up recovery from psoriasis and even help cancer patients cope better with the symptoms of both their treatment and their disease.[3]

It seems like every day there's a new study that's been published proving even more benefits of mindfulness. Launch an internet search on just about any mental health issue combined with the word mindfulness and you may find a new study that shows how mindfulness can help you in some very significant way. That's how potent mindfulness appears to be.

In this book, you'll not only learn the science behind WHY mindfulness works, you will learn how to use mindfulness in different ways, and for many different purposes. You'll learn how to use mindfulness to perform better at work, how to overcome insomnia and even how to cope better with chronic pain, anxiety, depression and issues with addiction. As you will see, mindfulness is an approach to life that you can practice every day. Every moment that you spend practicing it, can change your brain in positive ways that you will appreciate, more and more, as you begin to make the practices outlined in this book a daily habit.

I have a friend named Trish Meili. Trish and I had been in the same yoga class for about two years before I discovered that I had known of her for over 20 years. You probably know of her, too. This is how I found out: As we were leaving class one day, I said, "I'll see you next week."

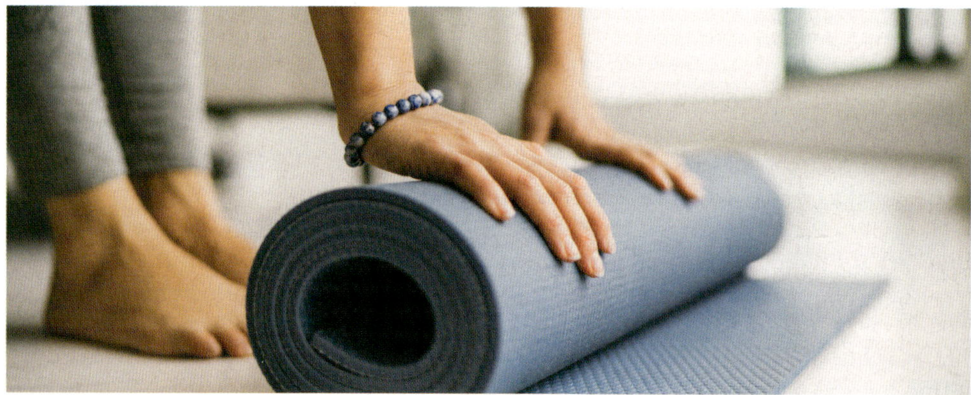

"No," she said. "Next week, I won't be here."

"Really? Where are you going to be?"

"Traveling."

"Doing what?"

"I'm giving a keynote speech at a conference in Hilton Head, South Carolina."

Trish was always so quiet and shy in class; I couldn't BEGIN to imagine her giving a speech to a large conference in a far-off place.

"What will you be speaking about?"

"My book."

"Wow, you wrote a book! What is it about?"

To my surprise, she hesitated a bit before telling me, as if she didn't really want me to know. She probably thought everyone in class knew who she was, but obviously I had no idea. And now that she realized I didn't know, there was no way to say what she was about to say next without leaving me in total shock.

"It's about how I was raped and beaten in Central Park."

That's when I learned that Trish Meili was much BETTER known as "The Central Park Jogger." Respecting her privacy, no one in the class had ever mentioned it to me before. She had taken up yoga and mindfulness to help herself recover from her injuries. A few months later, when I told Trish I was going on a 6-day mindfulness retreat with author and mindfulness expert Jon Kabat-Zinn, she casually said, "Tell Jon I said hello."

"You know Jon Kabat-Zinn?" If you Google Jon Kabat-Zinn, you will not only find a ton of You-tube videos, but you will also find his name cited in a lot of scientific studies on mindfulness. He is the author of many best-selling books on mindfulness and the Washington Post calls him "Mr. Mindfulness."

"Yes I know Jon," Trish said in her quiet way. "Practicing mindfulness was an instrumental part of my recovery. When I was in rehab Jon met me and offered to help."

"When I woke up in the hospital three weeks after the attack," she explained, "the last thing I remember was standing in my New York apartment thinking I wanted to go for a run in Central Park. I don't remember a single thing after that."

"I had no idea how bad my condition was until I was transferred to a rehabilitation hospital in Connecticut. At my first rehab session, the therapist held up a cardboard clock, used for teaching school children how to tell time. I knew I was looking at a clock, but I couldn't decipher what those hands meant. Apparently, that's not uncommon for people with traumatic brain injuries."

"I couldn't allow myself to get bogged down by this or any other discouraging news, like blaming others or feeling victimized. I had to forget the past (before the attack) and not worry about the future (what functionality I might or might not recover). I had to let all that go."

"I remember watching TV and seeing reports about ME in the news. Doctors who didn't even know me, and had never examined me, were making pessimistic predictions about my recovery. They would say terrible things like: She will probably never walk again, or talk again, or live a normal life. Somehow, I had to tune out all that noise. I did it with mindfulness. And Jon Kabat-Zinn helped me learn how to do this."[4]

A lot of this book is built around concepts I first learned during my 6-day retreat with Jon Kabat-Zinn. In the last chapter, I will share with you a day by day account of that retreat where we learned about informal mindfulness practice, formal mindfulness practice, present moment awareness, mindfulness exercises, and many different varieties of mindfulness meditation. All things you will learn about too, by reading this book.

Probably the most important thing I learned about mindfulness was something Jon Kabat-Zinn said on the very first night of that retreat. It would inspire me to *want* to change at a very deep level: "Awareness doesn't get depressed; Awareness doesn't get anxious; Awareness doesn't get angry."[5]

On one level, I had no idea what he was talking about. But, on another level, I really wanted whatever it WAS he was talking about. These were ALL issues, I had been dealing with to varying degrees, my entire life. If awareness could somehow help me deal with being depressed, anxious and angry, I wanted to do whatever it would take to get me there.

Body Scan

A classic Mindfulness-based Stress Reduction (MBSR) exercise which you can do in just one minute, is called body scan. This relaxation technique involves mentally moving through your body, point by point (from head to toe) and noticing any tension you might be holding at each point, and then consciously letting it go. You can do this exercise lying down or sitting in a chair. You can close your eyes or leave them open. Start by taking several deep breaths in and out.

Begin scanning at the top of the head. Notice your scalp area – if there is any tension there, let it go. Now notice the muscles in your forehead. We typically hold a lot of tension there. See if you can just relax that area. Move down to your jaw. Relax your tongue in your lower jaw. Let your jaw drop just slightly.

Now notice the muscles in your neck and shoulders. Lower your shoulders. Move down to your belly, see if you can let it expand out just a bit, relaxing any hidden tension you might be holding there. Notice any tension in the upper legs, your lower legs, and let it go. Now move down to your feet, letting any remaining tension in your body, flow right out through the tips of your toes.

The next morning at breakfast a psychiatrist told me about some promising research going on in Canada where mindfulness was being used to treat depression. He said that Dr. Zindel Segal was having great success using this method.

He went on to explain "each episode of depression increases the odds of another episode, by about 50%. That means someone who has suffered from two or three episodes of clinical depression is virtually untreatable. Treatment-resistant depression is one of the fastest growing mental health problems in the United States."[6]

Once you've experienced even one bout of depression, you WORRY about having another bout. So, every time a blue mood comes on, even for just a few hours or a few days, you're terrified that you'll relapse into another bout of clinical depression. Zindel Segal's work was addressing that very problem.

This information was very encouraging to me, and it helped me jumpstart my meditation practice. It would take several years of dedicated work, but eventually mindfulness, combined with a habit of regular exercise and healthy eating, would help stop, what at the time of the retreat, seemed like a never-ending battle with either depression itself, or the FEAR of relapsing into depression.

Now you see why I came back around to embracing mindfulness. Besides helping me avoid anger and worry, it also helped me deal with some pretty major issues like depression and anxiety. It helped my friend Trish recover from major head trauma. And as I have tried to illustrate, staying in the present moment has the potential to help us all overcome distractions, reduce errors and save time.

As I said earlier, studies show that mindfulness helps sufferers with eating disorders, addiction and chronic pain, not to mention the studies that show it can improve immune system functioning, speed up recovery from psoriasis, and help cancer patients cope better with the symptoms of both their treatment and their disease.[7]

All these amazing benefits can be yours for the taking. You just have to be willing to consider what Jon Kabat-Zinn said on that first night about awareness. There's a place, he would later explain, inside of every one of us, where this awareness resides. We just have to get in touch with it.

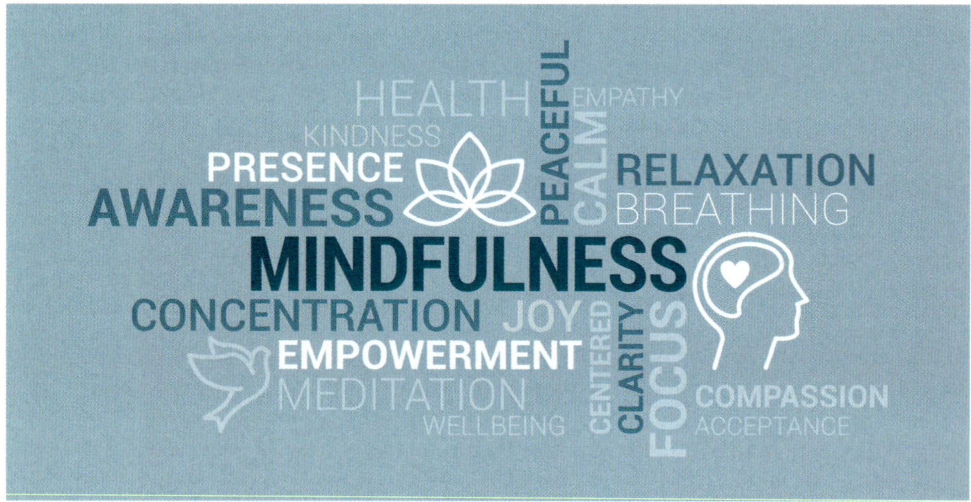

It's a place where we can observe our thoughts, our emotions and our moods – in a more objective and detached way. Psychologists call this ability to witness our thoughts and emotions: *distanciation*. The more we practice distanciation, the better we get at it.

As a culture, we tend to put the thinking mind up on a pedestal because the thinking mind has created so many wonderful things like skyscrapers and computers and great works of art. So, it wouldn't even occur to most westerners to WANT TO DISTANCE themselves from their thinking. But if you've ever criticized yourself unmercifully (or someone else) for making a stupid (or innocent) mistake, *you start to see how fallible the mind can be*. It pessimistically assumes the worst in difficult situations: about us, about our loved ones and virtually everyone we know.

That's one reason why we mistake *what we think with who we are*. When we say things to ourselves like, "I'm a terrible person," *we believe it*, even though we might not believe it if someone else said it. But the more we practice *distanciation* and the more we cultivate this awareness, the less power these negative, pessimistic and sometimes self-destructive thoughts have over us.

In order to get the full benefit of mindfulness we need to STOP making the mistake of believing those disturbing thoughts are true or who we are. They are not. We are the awareness that can observe those thoughts. That's what Jon Kabat-Zinn meant when he said awareness doesn't get angry, depressed or anxious.

This is an incredibly liberating idea. *But it may take reading this entire book before you even start to believe that.*

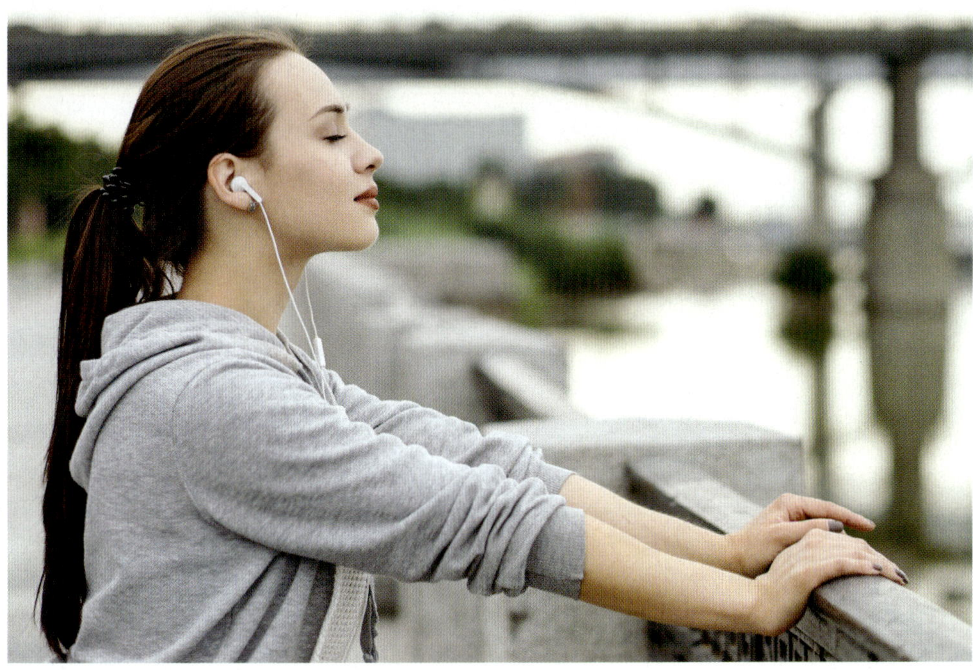

Chapter 2

Ten Easy Ways to Practice Mindfulness

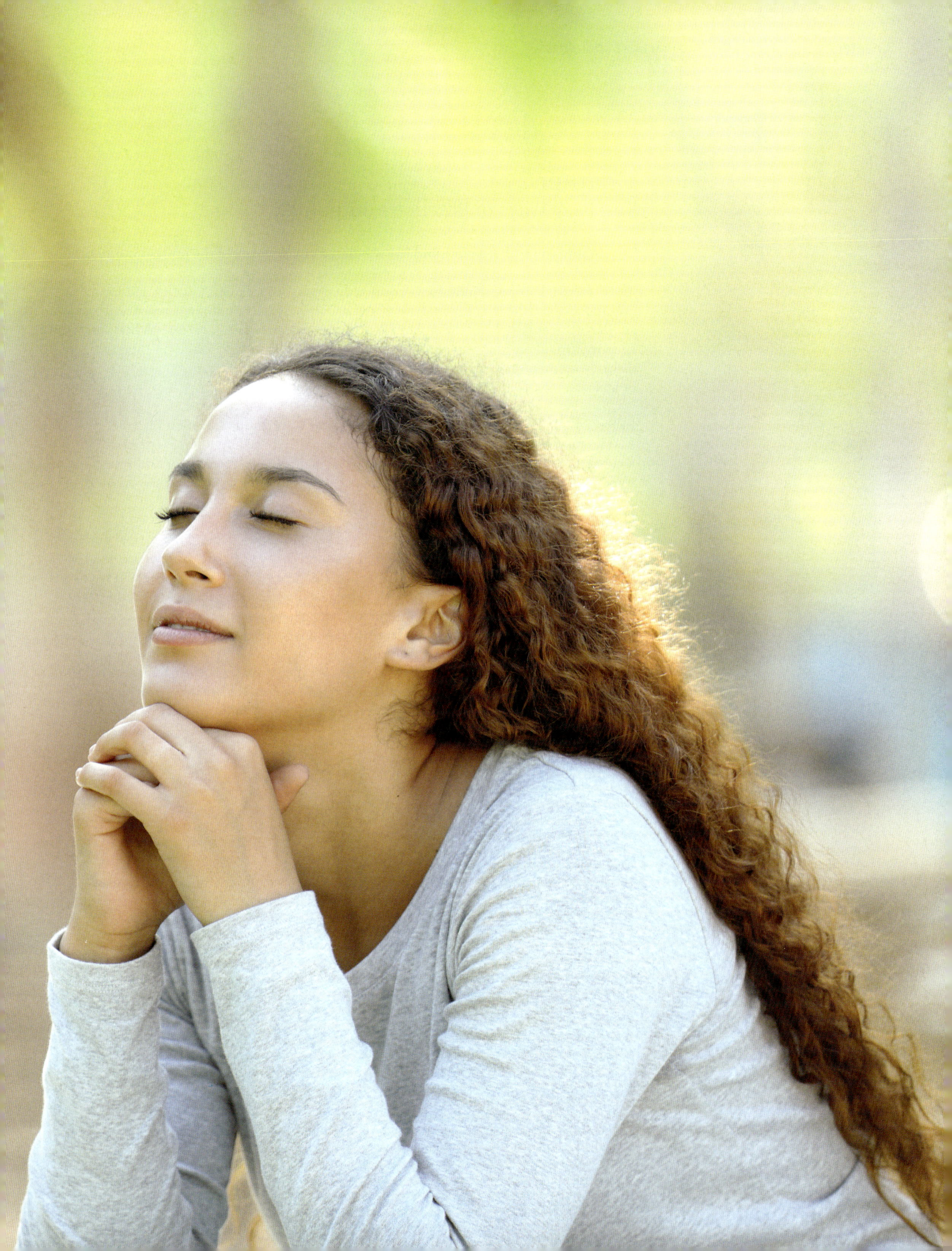

Chapter 2
Ten Easy Ways to Practice Mindfulness

The minute you realize your mind has wandered you are back in the present moment.

There are two kinds of mindfulness practice: Everyday mindfulness practice and formal mindfulness practice. In chapter 1 we talked about everyday mindfulness practice. These are the little things you do throughout your day to pay *attention on purpose*. When you keep your mind on what you are doing while you are doing it, like while washing the dishes, your mind moves away from ruminating on thoughts that might make you angry or anxious.

In formal mindfulness, you take time out to *practice* some form of meditation every day. Besides qualifying you for a long list of health benefits, formal mindfulness practice helps you fine tune your everyday mindfulness skills as well. For example, if you find your mind wandering a lot during the day, formal practice will help you learn how to stay focused on one thing at a time.

If you find yourself having trouble letting go of anxious or angry thoughts, formal practice will help you get better at releasing them. If you find that you startle easily or are quick to lose your temper, formal practice can help alleviate these issues as well. As we will see in chapter three, formal mindfulness practice changes the structure of your own brain. These changes in the brain explain why mindfulness can help us lower stress and anxiety, reduce depressive episodes and increase our levels of happiness.[1]

The most common formal mindfulness practice is called *breath awareness*. This form of mindfulness meditation is so simple, it's hard to believe that you are *doing* anything at all. But don't let that "simplicity" fool you. Directing your attention to your breathing in this way can be trickier than you think.

Just breathe

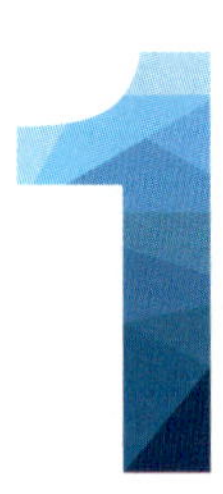

2-MINUTE MEDITATION #1

Breath awareness. Set a timer for two minutes. You probably have one on your smart phone. Sit in your chair, feet flat on the floor, hands in your lap while sitting up straight. Notice every in-breath and every outbreath. If your mind wanders away from your breathing, simply bring it back to noticing the breath.

Ironically, when you first sit down to meditate, instead of slowing down, sometimes your thinking mind speeds up and goes into overdrive. Like most Americans, you are probably not used to sitting still and doing nothing. It feels wrong. You feel like you should be doing something more constructive and less passive. But these thoughts are all just *judgments*. Mindfulness, to a large degree, is about *non-judgment*. And to become better at mindfulness you must *practice* non-judgment by first becoming aware of how often judgments play a role in your mood, your emotions and your thinking.

In the next exercise, which includes thought watching, look for any judgments that come up.

2-MINUTE MEDITATION #2

2

Breath awareness + Thought watching. Set a timer for 2 minutes. Notice your own breathing. Notice every in-breath and every outbreath. But this time, also notice any judgments that come up like: Why am I doing this? Or, I'll never figure this out; This is a dumb idea; And at the other end of the spectrum: This was easy. Maybe too easy. There's got to be a better use of my time.

You'd think everyone would take to breath awareness like a duck takes to water. Unfortunately, that's not always the case. We are easily distracted, one thought leads to another and many times, when that happens, you don't even realize that you're not really meditating any more.

This all-too common phenomenon is called **monkey mind.** Think of monkeys sitting in a tree, jumping from branch to branch. That's exactly what your mind loves to do. It jumps from one thought to another and on to another. Before you know it, you are LOST IN THOUGHT, totally unaware of your surroundings. *That's mindlessness.*

When this happens to a beginning meditator, the first thing you will notice is a lot of overly-negative judgments come up about your inability to meditate, sit still, or keep your mind focused on one thing at a time: All because of this innate tendency – that just about everyone has – toward mental fluctuation or monkey mind. This leads a lot of people to the false conclusion that *they are incapable of meditating*. This is one of the most common complaints of beginning meditators and what often causes them to quit, practically before they get started. One way to deal with this problem is to meditate on: *Not being judgmental about your own judgments.*

This sounds a little crazy but it's a key piece of the mindfulness puzzle. Every time we meditate, we can practice non-judgment. How? By *not judging ourselves* when we experience: mind-wandering, self-destructive thoughts, and most of all, *judging*. (So, don't judge the judging.)

2-MINUTE MEDITATION #3

3

Breath awareness Thought watching + Non-judgment. Set a timer for two minutes. Notice every in-breath and every outbreath. Also notice any judgments that come up. *I'm not good at this, this is too difficult for me, etc.* Try not to judge the judgments. Don't give them any power by judging them. Just watch them come and go, almost like you'd watch clouds rolling by and covering up the sun on an otherwise mostly sunny day.

Experts say the goal of mindfulness is not to try to change your thinking but to change your *relationship* to your thinking. Like we said in chapter 1, your thinking is not who you are. With the help of the three previous exercises, you can clearly see, the thinking mind likes to pass judgment on just about everything. Is this who you are? Are you super judgmental? Probably not, *but your thinking mind is.* Now you can begin to see what we mean when we say you are NOT your thoughts.

Sitting back and watching this tendency is positively therapeutic because it allows you to SEE that you can *choose* whether you want to believe a judgment (that your own mind has spun out) like: *I'm no good at meditating.* It also allows you to choose to go down an entirely different path with an entirely different outcome: *I can do this. I know I can. It will take some effort, but from the evidence I've read so far, it's truly worth the effort.*

This is a very empowering thought and it applies – not just to meditation - but to *just about every challenging aspect of personal growth, you may ever encounter.*

Other problems beginning meditators have are differentiating between:

1. When they are actually meditating and when they are not.
2. When they are *thinking* about their meditation and NOT *actually* meditating.
3. When they are lost in thought and when they have returned to meditating.

Let's say you decide to meditate on the sound of rain on the roof. (Yes, this is a form of mindfulness meditation.) At first, it's very relaxing. You can't believe how easy it is but that's when you realize, you're not meditating, *you're thinking about how easy it is.*

You eagerly go back to focusing on the sound of the rain. Again, you maintain your focus on the rain for a while, and again it's very relaxing. *This is just wonderful, you think.* Whoops, you say, there I go again, thinking about the meditation and not meditating. Maybe that's why experts like John Kabat-Zinn say over and over again that the goal of mindfulness is NOT to stop thinking. It's basically impossible for the average person to stop thinking. So, whatever you do, don't judge it when your mind wanders off: *Thinking happens.*

But here it's helpful to realize that when you are thinking about the rain in any way, while yes, that's different from *just listening to it,* your mind is still focused on what you are doing while you are doing it, so that's OK. It's when your mind wanders completely away from what you are doing, that it can be problematic: That's when you may begin to ruminate, consider self-destructive thoughts or hang onto and amplify disturbing emotions. Instead, you can just watch your mind wander, and not judge it.

2-MINUTE MEDITATION #4

Sonic meditation. Set a timer for two minutes. Find a quiet place where you won't be disturbed. Close your eyes and just notice the sounds within the room. Notice the sounds from the building you are in but outside the room. Now notice the sounds just outside the building or just outside your (perhaps open) window. See if you can even notice any sounds coming from far away. Notice whether you are *thinking* about what you are hearing or just truly *listening* to it. (If you hear your mind identifying different sounds, saying, "oh that's a bird and that's a cricket" you're probably *thinking* about the sound more than just taking it in.) And finally, notice if your mind ever wanders off the sounds you are hearing and onto something completely unrelated.

Some people don't feel comfortable closing their eyes when they meditate. If this is true in your case, you can relax your eyelids, so they are half-closed and stare at something that is not moving, or perhaps on the floor in front of you.

One of the most helpful things that Jon Kabat-Zinn said on my six-day retreat was this: "*The minute you realize your mind has wandered you are back in the present moment.*"

What you are trying to cultivate here is attention to what you are doing while you are doing it. So, when you think about how wonderful the meditation is, that's OK. But when your mind completely wanders off, and you start thinking about your to-do list, that's when you want to "wake up" and bring your attention back to the point of focus.

Having said that, it helps to know that your mind is *constantly* wandering off. And bringing it back to the point of focus, just like learning not to judge the judgments, is an integral part of mindfulness practice. Here again, we are learning an important skill every time we drag our minds back to the point of focus: Whether that point of focus is on your breathing, watching your thoughts or listening to the sounds in the room.

This attention-grabbing process is often compared to weight-training. Every time your mind wanders, just bringing it back, without judgment, is like doing reps at the gym. The more often you do it, the stronger you get. The same is true of bringing yourself back when your mind is lost in thought. It's an opportunity to get better at strengthening the mind's ability to focus on what you are doing while you are doing it.

2-MINUTE MEDITATION #5

5

Sonic meditation + thought watching. Find a quiet place where you won't be disturbed for two minutes. Close your eyes and just notice the sounds within the room. Notice the sounds nearby. Notice the sounds just outside the room. Notice the sounds from far away. Also notice when you are THINKING about your meditation and how that's different from just listening intently. Then notice when your mind wanders so completely that you are lost in thought. Whenever that happens – without judgment - bring your mind back to the point of focus.

OK, so hopefully you've noticed exactly what it means to be totally lost in thought and how that affects you when you are trying to meditate. But you also know that the minute you realize you are lost in thought *you are back in the present moment*.

One of the keys to understanding the difference between thinking about meditating and just meditating, is understanding the difference between thinking, doing and being. Deepak Chopra, a prolific author and mindfulness expert likes to say: "We are NOT human doings. We are not human thinkings. We ARE human beings." Yet we seem to spend just about ALL our time *thinking and doing*.

What does it mean to just be? And why would that be better than thinking and doing? And how will that help my meditation practice?

Thinking can be problematic. We've seen some of the downsides of wayward thinking already: Rumination, self-destructive thoughts, anxious thoughts and angry thoughts. But there's something else about thinking that only the mindfulness tradition seems to recognize: When we *think* about something, we are always a little removed from the action.

For example, when I go to a party where I don't know anyone, I find myself over-thinking that point and it separates me from the other people in the room. My thinking usually goes like this: "I don't know a single soul at this party. This is not my kind of crowd. Look at how differently everyone is dressed. I'm under-dressed. Maybe I should leave right now." Over-thinking things often keeps us in a bubble, separated from everybody and everything around us.

Doing is important but it has its downside too. Just like thinking, which at times can be very productive, doing has many important aspects, also. We wouldn't be where we are today without having spent plenty of time doing and accomplishing things. But many of us get so addicted to doing, we can't allow ourselves a moment's rest, or to sit still for as little as ten minutes and just be. Heck, we can't even allow ourselves to do one thing at a time. We must multi-task. Apparently, doing ONE thing at a time, just isn't good enough anymore. So, doing can keep us in a bubble too.

Being, on the other hand, can set you free. It will burst the bubble. Finding out what it feels like to just be, is one of the goals of mindfulness. An easy way to get there is to come to it through the portal of your five senses. Listening, feeling, tasting, smelling and really looking at the world around you, can all help bring you into the present moment and allow you to experience what it's like to JUST BE.

2-MINUTE MEDITATION #6

Feeling. Feel what it's like to sit in a chair. Notice all the places where your body touches the chair. Feel where your feet touch the floor. Notice anywhere the air touches your skin: On your hands, on your face, on the tip of your nose. Notice any breeze or air moving in the room. Notice any places on your body that are warm or cold. *Try to become one with those feelings.*

That last instruction: *Try to become one with those feelings,* and instructions like it, always used to annoy me to no end. When I first encountered mindfulness, it all seemed way too woo-woo to be of any use to me what-so-ever. But when I went on that six-day retreat, and we entered into the 36-hour "silent portion" of the retreat, I saw how addicted I was to thinking and doing.

The rules were simple: During that 36-hour period we were not supposed to read anything, look at TV, pick up our phones, use a computer or talk to anyone. We weren't even supposed to make eye-contact with one another. Because our meals were prepared for us, we didn't really have to do anything. And the minute you take away all those forms of distraction the only thing you *THINK* you have left to do is *thinking*. You also have being. But not everyone understands this at first or even what being means.

Half the people on the retreat HATED the silent part and the other half LOVED it. The part of the group that loved it, were forced by necessity, into figuring out how to just be. And what you discover when you focus on being over thinking and doing, *is that you can be happy with almost nothing at all.*

So, to *become one* with the feeling, or to become one with the *sounds in the room*, or to become one with the taste of the food in my mouth – these phrases that used to tick me off - now started to make sense. These are all ways of just being. Becoming one with anything is simply a pathway to being and it is a very pleasant alternative to the pain one often feels when one is trapped in one's own mind with nothing to do but just think.

2-MINUTE MEDITATION #7

Tasting. While often referred to as "the mindfulness raisin-eating exercise," you can do this activity with any small piece of dried fruit. A raisin has special qualities that make it especially appropriate for this exercise, but if you absolutely hate raisins (and it seems a lot of people do) try a craisin or dried strawberry or some other small piece of dried fruit instead.

Pick up the piece of dried fruit and hold it between your fingers. Think for a moment about where that fruit came from. Somebody, probably far away, had to pick it and then it was dried and packaged and shipped to a store near you.

Now mindfully examine the fruit in different ways: Roll it around between your fingers. Hold it up to your ear. As you continue to roll it between your fingers, you can often hear a barely perceptible sound. Now place it your mouth, but don't eat it. Roll it around between your tongue and the roof of your mouth. Carefully place it between your teeth but don't bite down. Not yet.

Notice any saliva building in your mouth and swallow that first. Now bite down. If you are eating a raisin you will get a tiny burst of flavor that seems much larger than you might expect from eating just one raisin. Now imagine what would happen if you ate all your food in this way. Would you savor it more? Do you think you might you eat less?

2-MINUTE MEDITATION #8

Listening. I love meditating on the sounds of nature: Rain on the roof, wind in the trees, crickets buzzing at nighttime, and birds chirping in the early morning. But my favorite natural sound, and one that for me, is super easy to meditate on, is the sound of a babbling brook. The next time you find yourself walking through a quiet park or hiking through the woods and you come to a secluded spot where you can sit by a stream, give this form of meditation a try. There's just so much to tune into, it's easy to *become one with the sound.*

2-MINUTE MEDITATION #9

Smelling. There is now a fair amount of research on the benefits of aroma therapy. And that has spawned an entire industry around providing people with all kinds of choices where aroma therapy is concerned. I personally like to keep a tiny pillow filled with pine needles next to my bed. I hold the little pillow up to my nose and take a few deep breaths. It really calms me down by instantly bringing me into the moment. A stress expert I know, Dr. Heidi Hanna, keeps a variety of aroma therapy bottles in her pocketbook. She says that different mixtures help her with different challenges.

2-MINUTE MEDITATION #10

Seeing. We are so accustomed to seeing things, without really *seeing* them, that eyesight doesn't always work as well as the other four senses do at locking us into the present moment. However, you *can* meditate using this sense, nonetheless. One pathway to the present moment is to simply stare at the flame of a candle. Another option is to close your eyes half-way and focus on the floor in front of you.

All these forms of mindfulness meditation have the potential to open YOU up to the special world of *just being.* That's one reason why these meditations are short, so you can make the adjustment from the distracted world of thinking and doing to the quiet world of just being. If you find that one of the above exercises, really strikes your fancy, try engaging in that one form of meditation for two minutes every day for one week.

Stanford University psychologist and behavioral change specialist BJ Fogg suggests that in order to establish a new habit, like a regular meditation practice, you have to make it so easy it requires almost no motivation at all. Finding a form of meditation that you can do for 2 minutes every day is a great way to create what Dr. Fogg calls a tiny habit.[2]

Fogg also suggests that you link your new behavior to an old habit that you already have in place like brushing your teeth. So, for example, a great time to start a meditation practice would be first thing in the morning.[3] Following Fogg's advice, you might say to yourself: Right after I brush my teeth every morning, I will meditate for 2 minutes. The new habit is easier to form when it rests on the back of a very reliable old habit that is already set in place. Focus first on forming the new habit. And once it's firmly in place, you can look to expanding it.

Compassion Meditation (Loving Kindness)

There is now a fair amount of research showing that compassion meditation has been proven effective in lowering stress reactivity, slowing down the aging process, increasing empathy and reducing inflammation after just 30 hours of practice. As long-time meditation teacher and author Sharon Salzburg teaches it, this meditation, which she calls Loving Kindness, is quite simple and easy to learn.

It's about meditating on: Wishing people peace and happiness, but it all starts with you and then works its way out to the larger community. It involves repeating silently (or quietly) to yourself, slight variations on the following sentence: May I be happy, may I be healthy, may I be free from suffering. You repeat this as many times as you wish. After wishing this for yourself, you then move out to the people in your immediate family: May my mother be happy, may she be healthy, may she be free from suffering, and so on.

Even if you don't like your mother, this prayer winds up helping you make peace with that fact. Thus, you can even do this loving kindness meditation with the names of people with whom you are having difficulties.

After that, you can work your way out to the entire community and the world around you, using more generalized terms. "May everyone in my town be happy, may they be healthy; may they be free from suffering." When you meditate on alleviating other people's suffering, it apparently frees you from thoughts of your own suffering, which can result in health benefits.

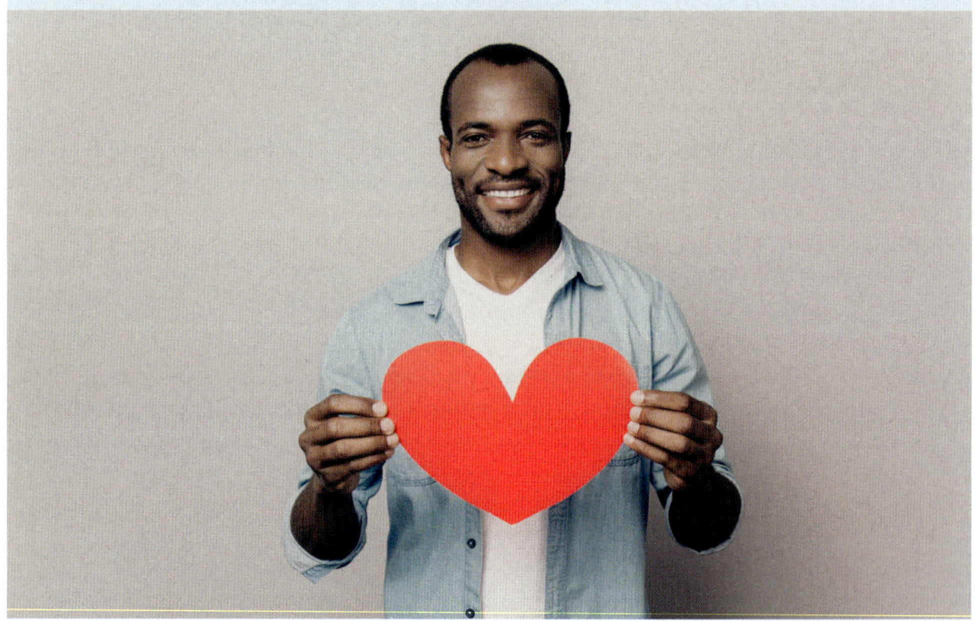

First you make your habits
and your habits make you.
Aristotle

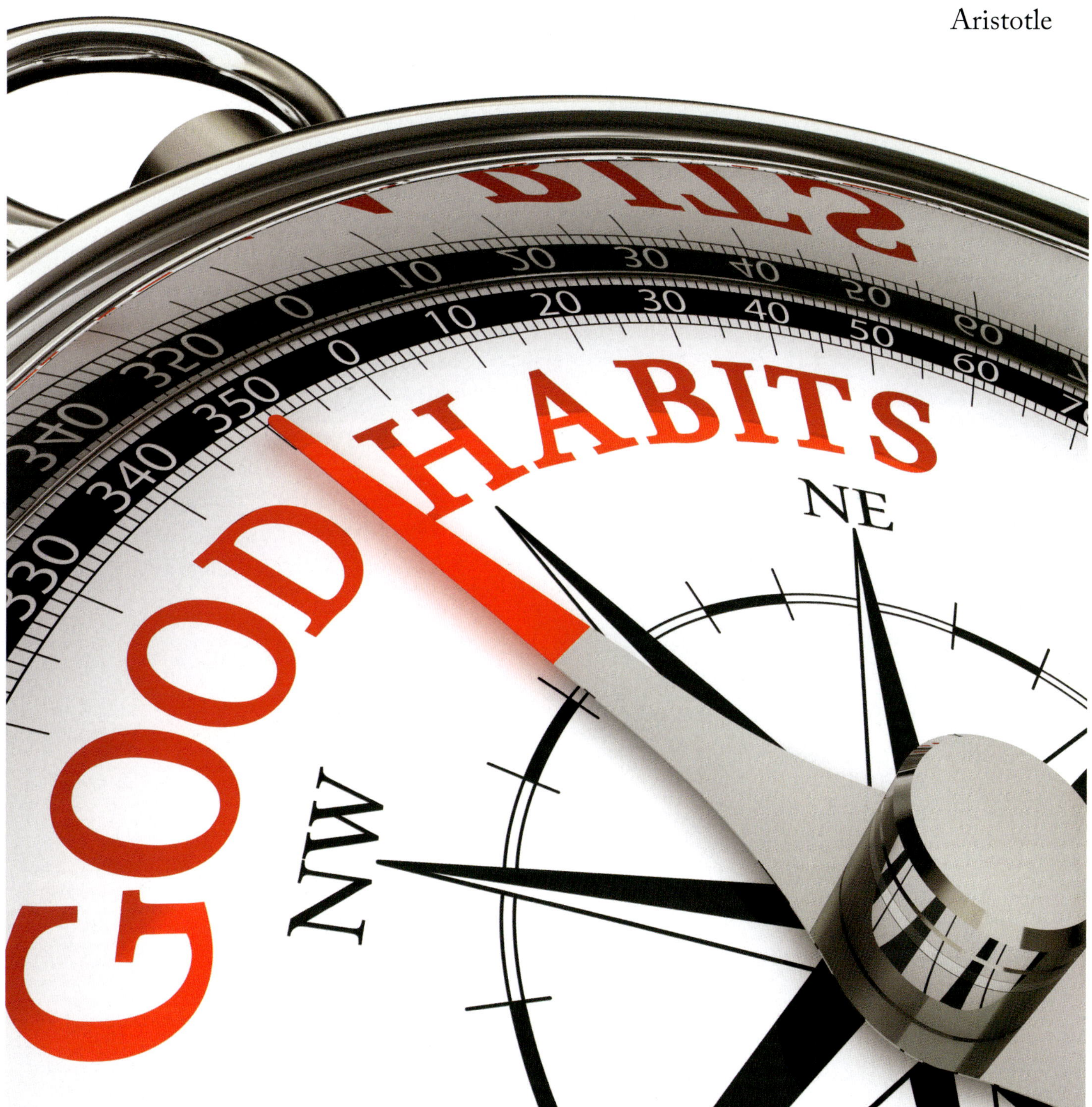

Chapter 3

The Science Behind Mindfulness

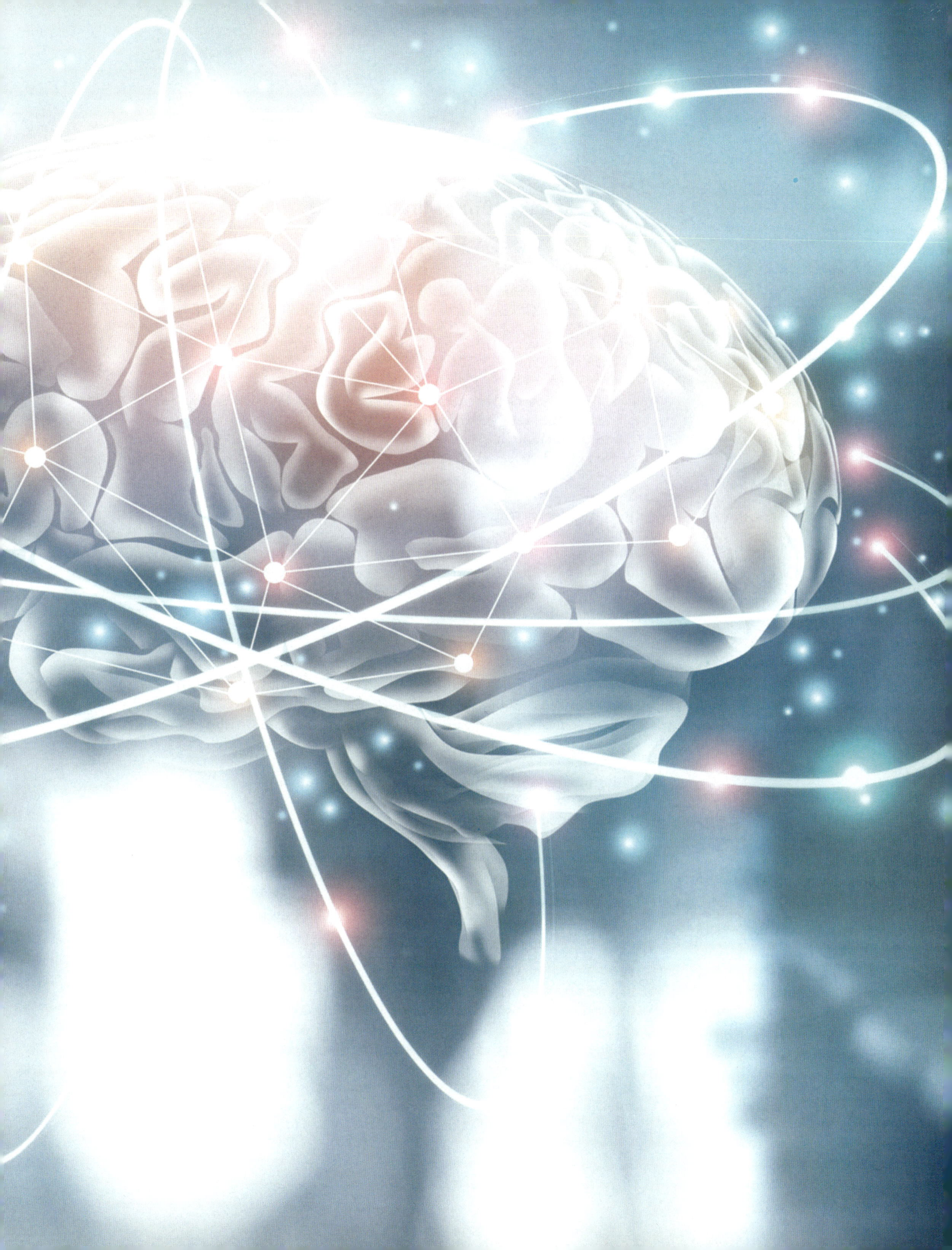

Chapter 3
The Science Behind Mindfulness

Trait effects vs. state effects

It was Dr. Ron Siegel, an assistant clinical professor at Harvard and author of the book, The Mindful Solution, who taught me the next most important thing I've learned about mindfulness: *The difference between state effects and trait effects.* State effects are what you feel *while* meditating. Trait effects are the lasting physical changes that occur as the *result* of meditating.[1]

Most people get into meditation for the state effects. Feeling relaxed, at peace, even blissful at times and one with the world are state effects. These feelings are all possible during meditation. But it's also possible for some people to feel no state effects at all, or even worse: To feel agitated or distracted. These folks usually give up on meditation rather quickly.

But if you fall into this second group, I wouldn't give up yet on the idea of meditating. Here's why: According to research by Sara Lazar, Ph.D., a Professor at Harvard University, whether you struggle with meditating or not, as long as you set aside time to do it, you can still get the benefit of TRAIT effects.[2] These effects include greater control over your emotions, sleeping better, reduced startle response, a boost in your immune system and, believe it or not, control over something that up until recently, science said could NOT be controlled by you: Your own genes![3] (More about that later.)

Over time, regular meditation can bring about an *increase* in size of the Prefrontal Cortex (or PFC), which is the command center of the brain. It can also cause the amygdala, where the stress response begins, to *decrease* in size. Every time you meditate, the higher areas of your brain are changing and growing and laying down new neural pathways that help you control the lower (more primitive) areas of the brain.[4]

Using mindfulness to change the structure of your brain.

Scientists used to believe that the brain stopped growing and changing at a very early age. This belief turned out to be entirely wrong. We now know our brains aren't fully developed until the age of 25 and continue to create as many as 10,000 new neurons *every day* right up until the day we die.[5]

If the brain didn't change throughout life, we couldn't function. Think about the last time you stayed in a hotel or spent a few days in an unfamiliar place. I know when I stay in a hotel where I've never been before, usually within minutes, I learn my way around the entire place. I figure out exactly where the restaurant, the vending machines, the elevator, and the fitness center are, and if I ever return to that same hotel, even years later, I can usually find my way back to those places with little or no difficulty whatsoever.

Brain scientists call this amazing ability to change the brain neuroplasticity.

If the brain didn't change in response to experience, we'd never be able to find our way through a city, or navigate a subway system or find something we put away over a year ago. And in more primitive times we'd never be able to find our way back home from a

Brain Science

Neuron
A brain cell.

Neuroplasticity
The brain changes in response to experience throughout our lifetime. Everything we learn, every good or bad habit we develop, and all the memories that are encoded in our neurons over the course of a lifetime, do so because the brain is malleable or plastic. It never stops changing until the day we die.

The Prefrontal Cortex (PFC)
The executive center of the brain. This is the area at the top front of the brain, right behind the forehead. It's the part of the brain that doesn't fully mature until age 25. Meditation can strengthen connections between this area and other important areas of the brain, improving our willpower and our ability to handle stress.

Post Cingulate Cortex (PCC)
When we get distracted, this is the part of the brain that becomes highly active. When we learn to quiet the PCC during meditation, we reduce mind-wandering, clinging, rumination, etc.

Amygdala
This almond-shaped area of the brain, found in the mid-brain, is responsible for vigilance and threat-detection. It's where the stress response begins.

Hippocampus.
Found right next to the amygdala, it's the area of the brain responsible for learning and memory. Chronic stress and Alzheimer's Disease will dramatically shrink this part of the brain. Meditation and stress reduction can restore it.

faraway hunt or back out to an important food source, like a fruit tree or a place where edible plants would grow in abundance. These are examples of neuroplasticity that help us to function better.

But your brain can also change in detrimental ways. Chronic stress has the opposite effect on the brain as meditation. It increases the size of the amygdala and decreases the size of the PFC. This is the downside of plasticity: If your stress is chronic, you can become *even more* sensitive to stress and have more difficulty handling it. As a result, you may develop a hair-trigger response to situations that challenge you, frustrate you or make you angry. *Unfortunately, plasticity can go both ways.*[6]

Dr. Elissa Epel, Professor at the University of California at San Francisco, agrees. In an article published on the American Psychological Association website entitled, "How chronic stress is harming our DNA," she explains: "Chronic stress wreaks havoc in the brain. It can cause neuroplastic changes that alter how we perceive and react to the world. Stress impairs our executive function (think PFC, here) which dampens our ability to resist impulses (think controlling the more primitive areas of the brain like the amygdala)."[7]

Richard Davidson, a professor at the University of Wisconsin, has been studying the brains of short-term and long-term meditators for years. He invites meditators from all over the world to his lab in Madison, Wisconsin to participate in these studies. Mindfulness meditation author Dr. Matthieu Ricard is one of those people. Dr. Ricard spends six months out of every year meditating full-time. Like a professional athlete, he has spent tens of thousands of hours honing his craft.

Back in Wisconsin, Professor Davidson can see changes that take place in the brains of meditators (both state effects and trait effects) with the help of an MRI scanner. Not only can he see these changes in real time (state effects) he can also measure some of the long-term results of meditation on the brain (trait effects). A lot of what we know about the benefits of mindfulness meditation come right out of Richard Davidson's lab. You will often find his name and Jon Kabat-Zinn's name on studies that have been published in medical and psychological journals.

Davidson can measure changes in the size of the prefrontal cortex (PFC) and he can measure changes in the size of the amygdala which is where the stress response originates. While Dr. Ricard was a remarkably calm person, Davidson wanted to scan the areas of the brain associated with calmness and stress and compare those with the same areas in non-meditators. When Davidson asked Ricard to slide inside his MRI machine, he could see that Ricard's brain was markedly different from the brain of an average person.[8] This was an interesting finding, but he needed more proof that meditation was the cause of these changes. So, he invited a dozen Tibetan Monks (who as part of their religious practice meditate up to eight hours every day) to his lab and studied their brains as well.

While in the MRI machine, the monks have no problem meditating what-so-ever. Don't forget, an MRI machine is a cigar-shaped tube that is so confining and makes such a loud banging noise, a lot of people panic at the prospect of getting inside one. Davidson asks the monks to not only relax in this confining space but to meditate on and off for 90 seconds at a time. When he observes the brain-scans of the monks in his lab what he sees is remarkable. The difference between when the monks meditate and when they stop meditating, *is like the difference between night and day.* "Entirely different

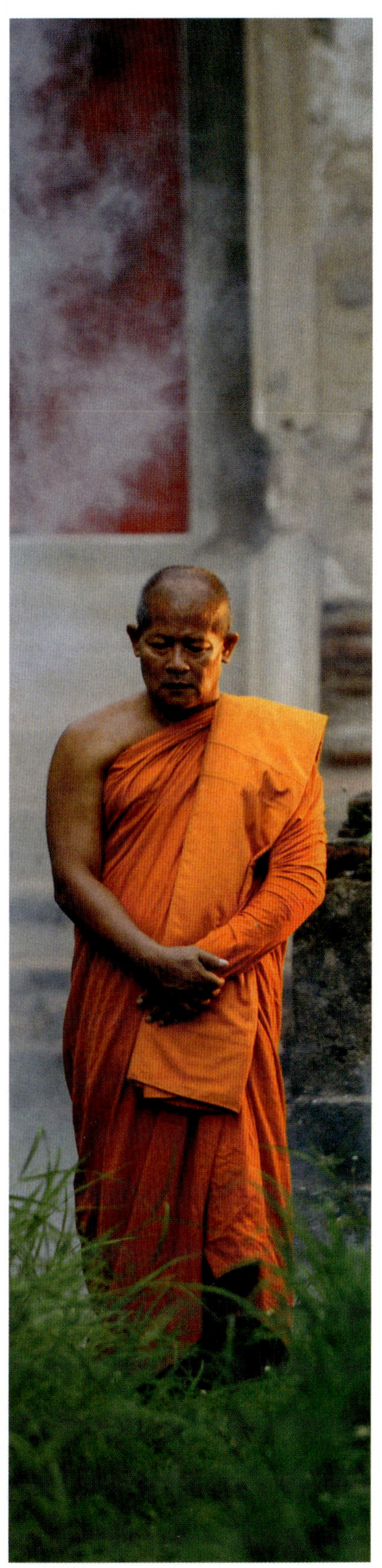

What's the difference between meditation and sleep and why can't I meditate lying down?

A sleep state is very different from a meditative state. When you're sleeping, for much of the time, you're unconscious: The lower more primitive parts of your brain (the hypothalamus and your brain stem) are running the show. When you're meditating, you're conscious: The more advanced part of your brain (the prefrontal cortex) is running the show.

When you get good at meditating, you are learning to use this advanced part of your brain to self-regulate your entire body down to a relaxed state that (in terms of brainwaves) is similar to a light sleep. But because you're awake, this is usually experienced as a delightful meditative state, entirely different from sleep.

When you're meditating, you're practicing how to concentrate and single-pointedly focus on one thing and one thing only, whether it's your breathing, the sounds in the room or repeating a mantra. This practice may eventually give birth to positive changes in the very structure of your brain. When you are asleep you are not practicing anything at all.

Continued on page 27.

areas of the brain light up. And it takes place the second they make the shift between meditating and not meditating."[9]

Davidson is literally seeing (and recording) *state effects* happening in the brains of these meditators. But more importantly, he can also measure changes in the size of different areas of the brain. That's when he sees *trait effects*. On average, Davidson reports, the difference in size between the PFC's of the monks compared to non-meditators is dramatic.[10]

With more of a thickening of gray matter in the PFC – considered the executive center of the brain - it's not surprising that these Tibetan monks have demonstrated unusual powers of self-control.[11] They can do things – in terms of self-regulating internal states – that the rest of us couldn't even dream of doing. The following passage, excerpted from the Harvard Gazette, describes what Harvard Professor and author of The Relaxation Response Herbert Benson, M.D. saw as he observed a demonstration of a meditation technique that Tibetan Monks practice called g Tum-mo:

> In a monastery in northern India, thinly clad Tibetan monks sat quietly in a room where the temperature was a chilly 40 degrees Fahrenheit. Using a technique known as g Tum-mo, they entered a state of deep meditation. Other monks soaked 3-by-6-foot sheets in cold water (49 degrees) and placed them over the meditators' shoulders. For untrained people, such frigid wrappings would produce uncontrolled shivering.
>
> If body temperatures continue to drop under these conditions, death can result. But it was not long before steam began rising from the sheets. As a result of body heat produced by the monks during meditation, the sheets dried in about an hour.[12]

This excerpt helps illustrate the difference between trait effects and state effects. Presumably, these monks felt a sense of inner calm while meditating. That's a *state effect*. But these monks also have extraordinary powers of self-control and self-regulation that is powered by a lifetime of meditating. *These are trait effects.* You probably won't ever need, or be able to dry sheets dipped in cold water on your bare back on a cold day, but you may, with just a modest practice, establish certain other *trait effects* that are just as important to you, like being able to gain control over fluctuating moods and disturbing emotions.

Until quite recently, the entire scientific world believed that your genetic make-up was set in stone from the day you were born. Whatever genes you inherited from your parents you were stuck with for life. This meant being genetically predisposed to whatever health problems your parents had. If one of your parents had heart-disease, cancer, diabetes or depression, you were more likely to have it too.

Now thanks to the emerging field of epigenetics, that belief is changing. The genes we inherit from our parents aren't the last word on how our bodies develop and change over time. We now know that certain genes have an on or off switch, called an epigenetic marker. Where we live, what we eat, whether we smoke or not, how much stress we experience, and believe it or not, *whether we meditate can determine whether certain genes get turned on or off.*[13]

Sugar consumption combined with stress can turn on genes for diabetes. Chronic inflammation can turn on markers for a whole host of other health problems.[14] There are even genes for how well we deal with stress that are found in the part of the brain (the hippocampus) responsible for learning and memory. Studies of rats (whose brains are roughly similar to humans) show that when a baby rat gets lots of licking and grooming in the first two weeks of life, the epigenetic marker for this particular anti-anxiety gene is turned on. And once turned on this gene, stays on for life.[15]

In the classic battle between nature (genes) and nurture (your upbringing and your environment) this is one place where nurture wins. While we can't change our upbringing, we can affect our epigenetic make-up by how well we take care of ourselves, including taking time out to meditate. And according to studies done in Richard Davidson's lab, health-enhancing epigenetic changes start occurring from the minute we start meditating. That data makes an even stronger case for the benefits of *trait effects*.[16]

There are four important takeaways from this chapter:

1. Understanding the difference between state effects and trait effects. State effects are what you feel *while* meditating and trait effects are the changes that take place over time, mostly in the brain, as the *result* of meditating.

2. Even if we struggle with meditation, we still get a health benefit from trait effects. As long as we set aside time to do it, everyone benefits from meditation. (20-30 minutes each day is ideal, but any amount can be helpful.)

3. Meditation changes the brain. By increasing the size of the prefrontal cortex and decreasing the size of the amygdala, meditation literally changes the form and function of our brains. These functional changes often result in reduced startle response, fewer anger episodes, greater control over a broad range of emotions, less depression, better sleep, and a boost in immune system functioning.[17]

4. Epigenetics. Perhaps the most impressive benefit of all is the ability to influence how your genes are expressed (turned on or off) by lifestyle choices. A healthy lifestyle that includes a regular period of meditation may make it possible for you to avoid (or dramatically postpone) certain lifestyle diseases marked by chronic low-grade inflammation such as heart disease, diabetes, arthritis and possibly even cancer.[18]

Most people in America don't get enough sleep. As you start to relax into meditation, you may also start to yawn and feel sleepy. If you meditate sitting up, typically you will wake yourself up if your head begins to nod. If you are lying down, you typically just fall asleep. That's why most meditation teachers discourage you from meditating while lying down. But if you don't fall asleep while meditating lying down, or if you want to USE your meditation to help you fall asleep, there's no problem with meditating while lying down whatsoever.

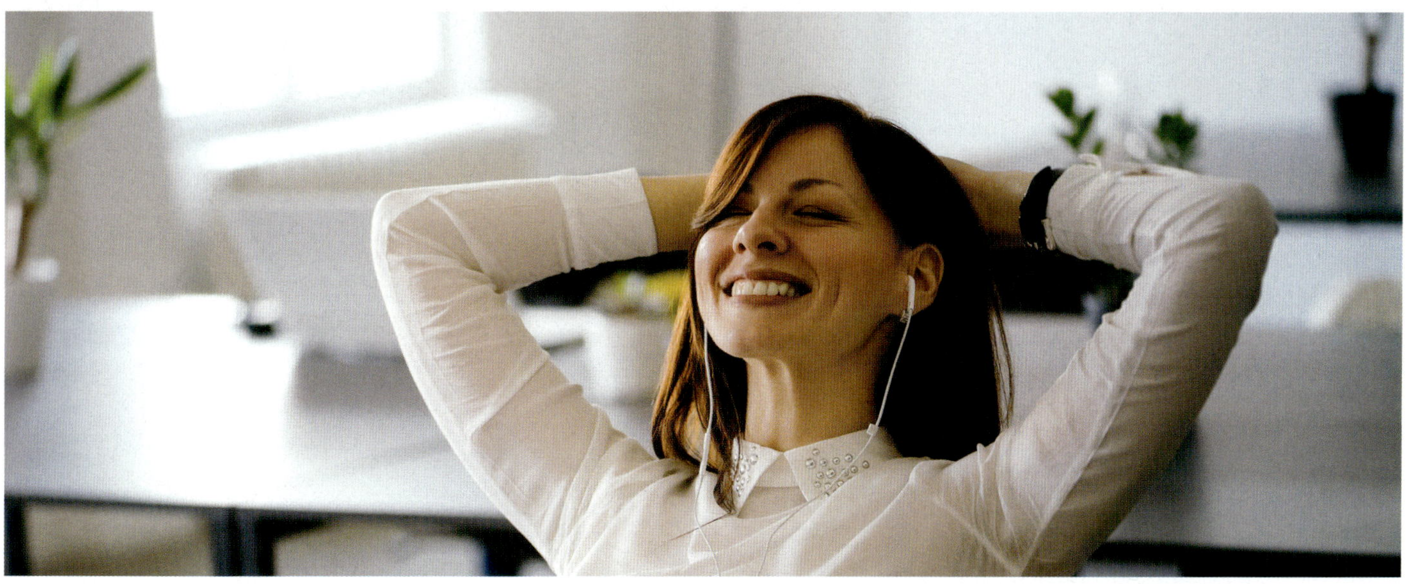

Chapter 4

Ten Mindfulness Techniques You Can Use at Home or On The Go

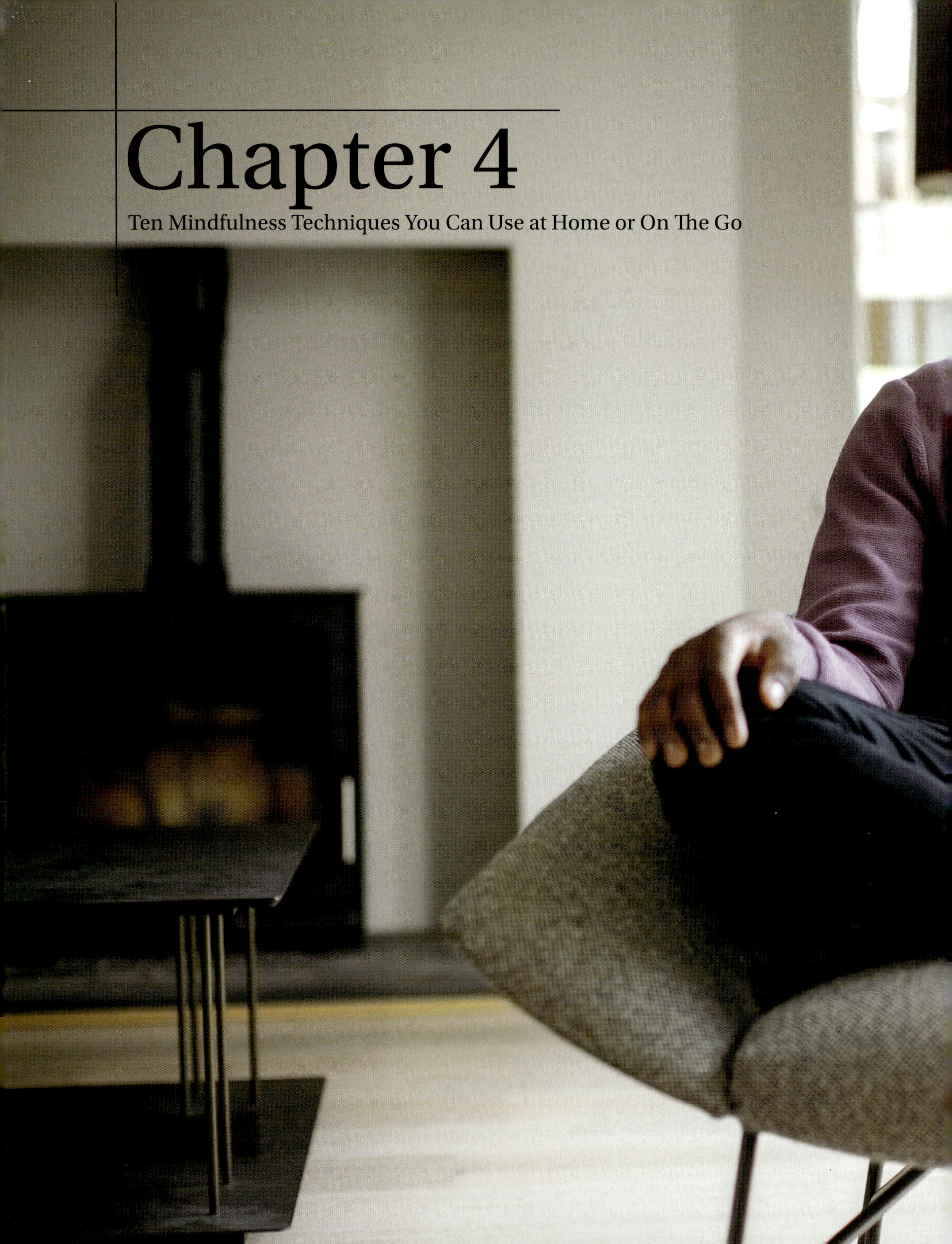

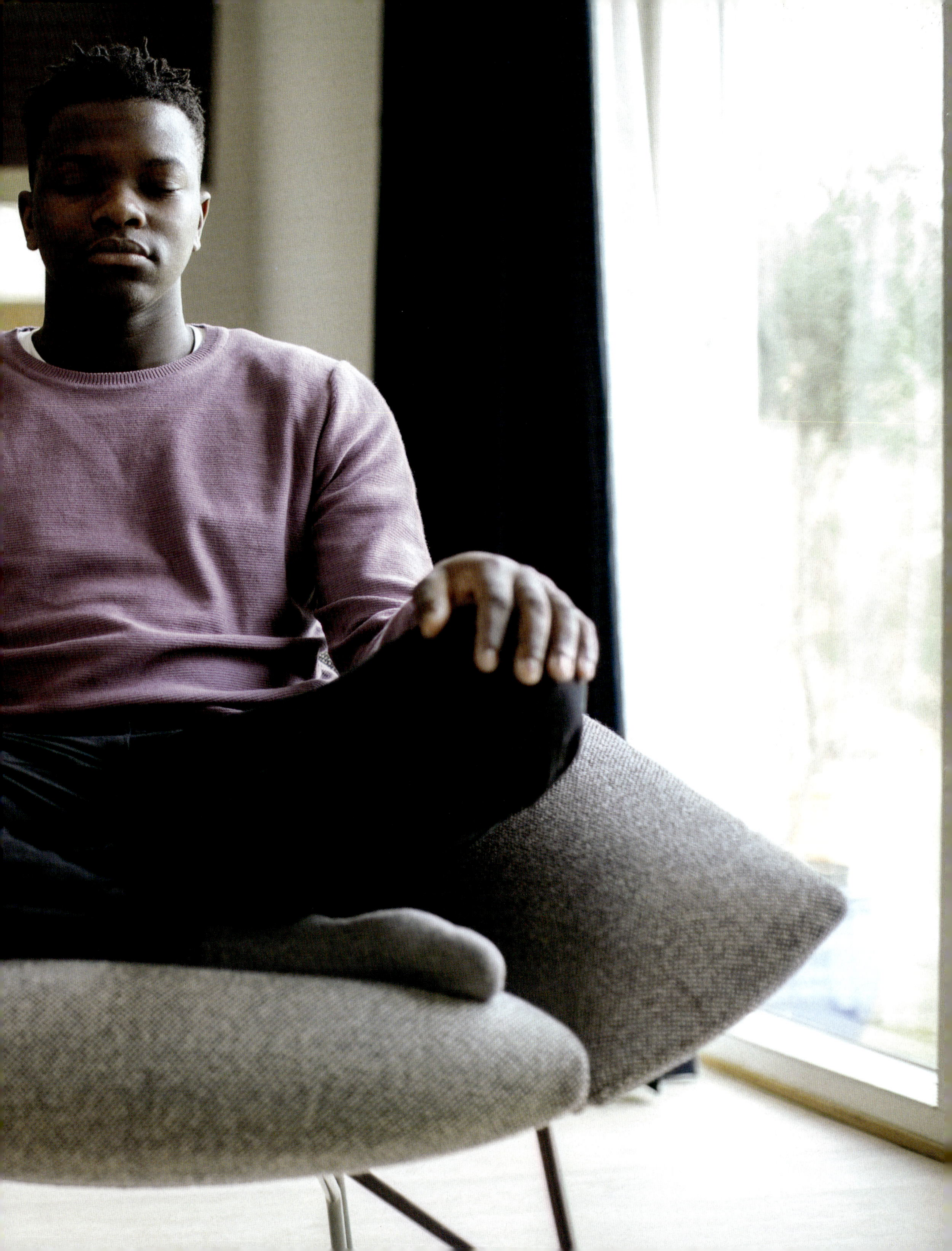

Chapter 4
Ten Mindfulness Techniques You Can Use at Home or On The Go
"I'll be happy when ..."

If you've ever worked out on a stationary bike, or just about any exercise device, you know that a lot of these machines can track all kinds of data from your heart rate to the number of calories you burn. Fifteen years ago, when I first joined a gym, I was tracking the calories I burned. I was aiming for an aspirational goal of burning 500 calories in 30 minutes. Bit by bit, I worked up from 300 calories in half an hour to 400. Each day, I would get on the bike and by riding a little faster, or setting the resistance a little higher, I'd move closer and closer to my goal. But for some reason, I just couldn't get over the 500-calorie mark no matter how hard I tried.

That's when I decided to try positive thinking. At first, I tried giving myself a little pep talk. "You can do this," I would say to myself before getting on the bike. "You've got this. You can do anything you set your mind to." I was hoping *positive thinking* would get me to my 500-calorie goal.

Trouble is, I've always been a bit suspicious of positive thinking. It sounds to me a bit like the gym teachers I had in high school, and the posters they would hang on the locker room walls: "There's no substitute for hard work." "Never wish life was easier, wish that you were better,"These posters were always quoting people I never heard of like Jim Rohn or Knute Rockne. I never really believed these posters so why should I believe myself when I sounded exactly the same way?

That's when I decided to try cognitive restructuring. Rather than putting on a phony-sounding positive voice, I attempted to do battle with my overly-negative thinking, which right around then was saying that this 500-calorie goal was *impossible.* Using cognitive restructuring, the voice in my head was now taking a different tack. It was saying: "When you first did 350 calories in 30 minutes, and then 400 calories in 30 minutes, you thought those goals were impossible, too. You passed those milestones a long time ago. Now you burn 450 calories without any problem. Why should 500 be any different?"

Cognitive restructuring is completely different from positive thinking, although many people confuse the two. Cognitive restructuring is always attempting to sort out the truth in a situation. Positive thinking will often try to sugar coat the truth, or rewrite the truth, which is why it can come off sounding phony. When you get fired or you find out you have cancer, or that there's a pandemic coming, positive thinking can sound more hopeful than believable.

Cognitive Restructuring never tries to stretch the truth. It simply tries to stop you from being OVERLY- negative. That's why sorting out the truth in this situation was important for me to do. My goal was aspirational, but it wasn't necessarily *impossible.* The truth is, I'd thought the previous milestones of 450, 400 and 350 had all been impossible, too. *But they weren't.*

One of the important things I started to do to attain each of the previous goals was to figure out exactly how fast (and at what resistance setting) I needed to pedal in order to achieve each of those three previous goals. Just maintain this speed for thirty minutes, I'd say to myself, and you'll make it. But when I got to the 500 calorie goal, I could keep up the pace for about 25 minutes or so and then I'd start to peter out and say it's *impossible* again and I'd feel myself run out of gas and miss the 500 mark by 25 or 30 calories.

That's when I decided to try mindfulness. This time around, I decided I would listen closely to my own body and see how tired IT was, rather than listen to my head saying how tired *I was*. Doing this I noticed that while I would get a bit winded toward the end, my core and my legs *were not tired at all.* I also noticed that I was more psychologically tired at the end than physically tired. One more thing I noticed with this mindfulness approach, was that if I burned some extra calories at the beginning, I'd be able to keep going at the end at a slightly slower pace, rather than giving up completely.

Once I put this whole mindfulness package together, that's when I started to get closer and closer to my 500-calorie goal. The most important thing I realized by the time I achieved the goal, was that my mind wanted to quit, but my body was up for the challenge. Noticing that subtle difference between the two, made all the difference in achieving my goal.

There are lots of practical ways you can use mindfulness in your everyday life to function better, feel better, achieve goals and be happier. Many of these mindfulness concepts have names like: "I'll be Happy When," "Name it and Tame it," "Impermanence" and "How am I doing Right Now?," which, as you will see below, is exactly what I used to get to my 500 calorie goal.

1. How am I doing right now?

1

There are many situations where this little mindfulness hack comes in handy. You can use it when you wake up in the middle of the night and your mind is all a twitter about something going on the next day or the next week. When you ask yourself this all-important question, usually the answer is quite calming: "*At this moment, I'm in a warm bed, it's comfortable and there's nothing that could possibly harm me right now.*"

I used a version of this question to get me over the hump of my 500-calorie goal. I slightly reworded the question to say: "How is *my body* doing right now?" I also used this question to get me through the Great Recession of 2008 and 2009 and the pandemic of 2020. Even though I was worried about my business failing on both occasions, I'd say to myself: Right now, I have enough money to get myself and my family through this day, this week and this month, I won't worry about it today, but I will take any steps I can undertake now that might improve my situation tomorrow, next week and next month.

Think of a situation you've encountered recently where asking this question might have helped you get through a difficult time:

____
____
____
____
____

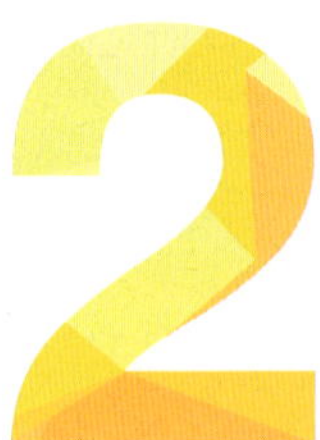

2. Name it and Tame it.

Most people don't like feeling stressed. We try to brush off the stress symptoms we are feeling inside. This may be one reason why so many people have issues with anxiety, anger, fear, and depression. Rather than acknowledging what it is that's bothering them, they try to cover it up and pretend it's NOT a problem. This strategy often backfires. As a result, unaddressed problems often grow larger and larger until they become debilitating.

Name it and tame it helps you acknowledge the issue in a variety of gentle ways that allow you to keep going without so much angst. Whenever you feel a strong emotion rising inside of you, *name it*: Wow look at how anxious am I about this. Look at how angry this is making me. Look at how frustrated I'm getting. Look at how fearful I am getting.

By NOT sweeping these feelings under the rug, you have a variety of choices. You can work with your self-talk to diminish these unwanted emotions: "These *feelings* are triggered by *thoughts* which I can control. Or, these are just feelings, and sometimes if I watch the feelings long enough, in a detached way, I will feel them subside. Or, you can *choose* to do something proactive, *in spite* of your feelings of fear, anxiety or frustration. Sometimes just taking one step – in the right direction - toward solving the problem, *dissolves the feeling*. That's how elegantly name it and tame it can work.

Think of a situation where you might be able to use Name it and Tame it:

____

____

____

____

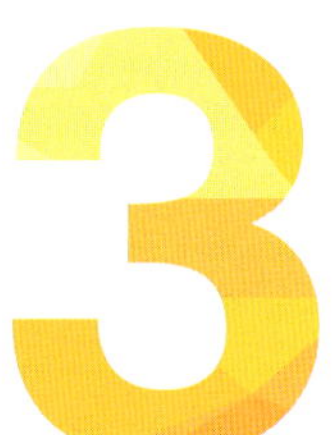

3. Beginner's mind

Seeing the world around you through the eyes of a child is often called: *beginner's mind*. Part of the reason we do so many things mindlessly, is that the world around us no longer seems new. But when we see things afresh, *with beginner's mind*, everything can seem new again. Think about how a child sees a cow or an elephant at the zoo, or snow or a beach for the first time. They are amazed by these sights. But for adults, it's just another meaningless thing.

But when you see the world with beginner's mind you look for aspects (about the same old thing) that you've never noticed before, whether it's that fresh shade of green you only see in the early spring, or an unusual cloud formation in the evening sky or the pleasurable taste and the crackling sound of a crisp apple as you bite into it. *There are infinite possibilities when you set your mind to looking at the world with beginner's mind.*

For years, whenever my wife and I went on a long trip, I would drive. I wanted to have something to do, to alleviate the boredom. Not only would I offer to drive, I'd bring a podcast or an audio book to listen to as well. Now, we share the driving so I can sit in the passenger seat and practice beginner's mind. As we travel through the countryside, often on deliberately chosen – slightly slower - back roads, I scan the horizon for anything I might not have seen or noticed before. All of the sudden, the whole world seems a LOT more interesting, and I really enjoy sitting in the passenger seat, a whole lot more.

What are some ways that *beginner's mind* might help you see an old situation (maybe even a recurring problem) in a whole new way:

____
____
____
____

4. I'll be happy when

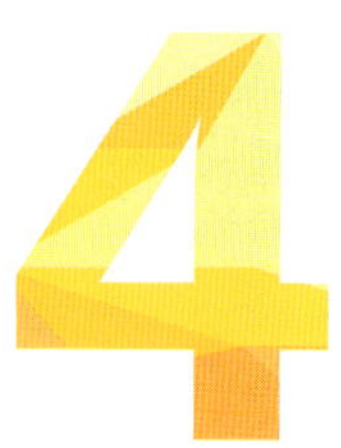

This is a soul-sucking habit that we all engage in. Usually it goes something like this: I'll be happy when I get a new boyfriend. I'll be happy when I get a new car. I'll be happy when I get that promotion. I'll be happy when I retire. I'll be happy when I get a new coat. I'll be happy when I make more money. *I'll be happy when I finish writing this book!*

Unfortunately, many of us feel we can't be happy until we get something, buy something, or accomplish something that we really want. When we finally do get THAT something, we are only happy for a short period of time until a NEW THING comes along that we want even more. With this mode of thinking our whole life goes by while we WAIT to get to a place where we are truly happy.

This *I'll be happy when* thinking is so pervasive it often goes by the name "the hungry ghost." It's the endless desire that follows us around like an insatiable ghost, always wanting more and never satiated for very long.

Make a list of three "*I'll be happy when*" examples that are holding you back from being happy right now.

1. ______________________________
2. ______________________________
3. ______________________________

5. Suffering

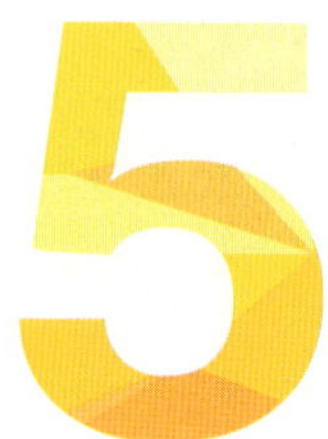

In the teaching of mindfulness, suffering is considered an innate characteristic of living. We all suffer. No one, no matter how well off, is immune to it.

All you need do is look at the royal family of England, to realize that even when you have everything you could ever want in life, you still suffer *royally*. Queen Elizabeth's father King George, who had a severe speech impediment, suffered because he NEVER wanted to be king. His older brother, who was in line to be king and wanted to be king, suffered too, because he also wanted to marry a divorced woman and had to give up the crown in order to do so.

King George's shy daughter, Elizabeth, didn't want to become queen but Margaret, her out-going younger sister, desperately did. Both suffered as a result of not getting what they wanted. And this only scratches the surface of the suffering that went on (and continues to go on) in that family.

Death, divorce, illness and pain are all part of the human condition. But so are the little moments of suffering like not getting a promotion, having someone tell you no, or having a friend not show up for a date. Sometimes we suffer when we should – by all rights – be having a wonderful time.

I remember this happening to me on a four-day trip I took to Martha's Vineyard. It was late June, and the weather was picture perfect each day: Sunny, not too hot, but still warm enough to swim. The water was unusually warm for that time of year, too. On the way over, I was happy as a clam, looking forward to my time on the island. The ferry ride was spectacular, and the scenery on the way over was beautiful. Four days later, on the ferry ride back, I was miserable. It was the exact same ride, with the exact same weather, and the exact same scenery, but I was clinging desperately to the events that had just transpired. I didn't want my perfect little vacation to end.

There was no way to stop time, so I suffered. This is one of the fundamental principles of mindfulness. Everyone suffers: In big ways and small ways. This leads to the three most basic principles of mindfulness:

1. There is suffering.
2. Clinging (or attachment) is the cause of suffering.
3. Letting go of clinging (or attachment) relieves suffering.

On the return ferry ride I was suffering because I was desperately clinging onto the past. But how in the world do you let go of clinging in a situation like this, or any situation in which you are suffering? We will discuss that in the next example. For now, think of three small ways, in which you might have suffered similarly:

1. ______________________________
2. ______________________________
3. ______________________________

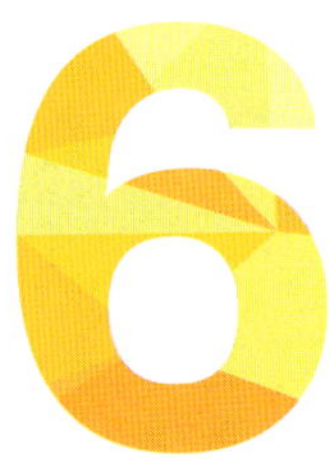

6. Non-attachment

Much of our suffering comes from attachment (or clinging) to how things were and can no longer be: Kids grow up, friends move away, money gets tight, relationships end, vacations end, and circumstances change. We lose things, we break things, a loved one dies, a child moves away, and downsizing occurs. This is the nature of life.

To the degree to which we become attached to these things, is the degree to which we suffer when they are gone. I used to have a subscription to a newspaper I dearly loved. Every morning, I'd walk to the end of the driveway and there it would be, waiting for me. Getting that paper, and reading it first thing every morning, made me feel great. When our money got tight, the newspaper had to go. But that's not the only thing we had to eliminate: We had to sell our home in what was becoming a trendy (but pricy) neighborhood. Taxes were going way up, and we needed to economize there too.

In both cases, I miserably *clung* (or remained attached) to these and other vestiges of what would soon be, my *former* life. But interestingly, once they were gone, I didn't miss them at all. A week after the newspaper stopped coming, I realized I had more time for other things AND I didn't have a huge stack of old newspapers lying around, waiting to be read. When we finally left the house in that pricy neighborhood for a less expensive house, I quickly realized what a huge psychological payoff it was to be able to *afford* the house we were living in.

Name three things that you are clinging to that are causing you to suffer:

1. ______________________________
2. ______________________________
3. ______________________________

7. Attraction and Aversion

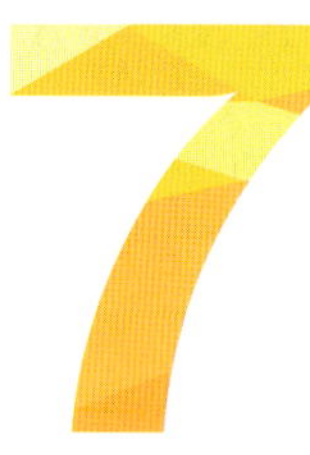

Something that you start out loving will often be something that you wind up hating. This happens with cars, clothes, apartments, houses, jobs and even relationships.

Sometimes it takes years, sometimes weeks and sometimes it happens in a matter of hours: Ever bought something at the mall, and by the time you get it home, you hate it? Salespeople know all about this. This all-too-common change of heart is called *buyer's remorse.* Every high-end salesperson is taught specifically how to guide a customer through buyer's remorse, so the customer doesn't try to return the item for a refund.

Watch out for attraction and aversion. Sometimes it happens with the things you love most: Your favorite coat, now with an imperceptible stain on it becomes your least favorite coat. A cool cell phone that you once loved, suddenly gets a noticeable scratch on it, and now you hate it every time you see that scratch. It's an interesting (and fairly common) phenomenon and most of us are barely even aware how frequently it affects us.

List three things you once loved that you now don't care for, or even dislike:

1. ______________________________
2. ______________________________
3. ______________________________

8. Impermanence

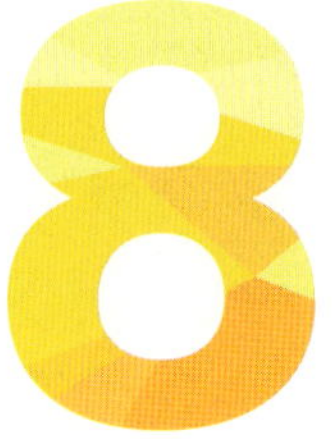

Sometimes referred to as the law of impermanence, mindfulness teaching recognizes that everything changes, all the time. Yet, we live our lives as if this rule was exactly the opposite: That everything always remains the same, *or at least it should.*

This too shall pass, is a saying that applies to all things good and bad. So, if you are caught in a down cycle where you are suffering – not to worry - *this too shall pass.* If you are currently in an up cycle, don't get too attached to it, because *this too shall pass.* If you are in pain now – that pain is going to fluctuate, and in most cases, *completely subside.* Happiness will pass, but grief will pass also. Nothing is permanent, not even granite, which changes imperceptibly over time.

In order to avoid suffering, we simply need to let go of the notion that we will always be happy and equally embrace the notion that we WON'T always be sad. If we fully adopt the idea of impermanence: we are embracing a fundamental, universal truth. *This too shall pass.*

List three things that would be made better right now by embracing the law of impermanence on the following page.

1. ______________________________
2. ______________________________
3. ______________________________

9. I, me, mine.

The last song *ever recorded* by the Beatles was, "I, Me, Mine," written by George Harrison. George was getting into meditation and spirituality at the time and he was seeing these three words popping up, repeatedly, in his reading. He understood that I ME MINE was a metaphor for ego and its potentially destructive force. He had experienced this force firsthand watching John Lennon and Paul McCartney (along with John's wife Yoko Ono) fighting constantly over who was the true leader of the band and who should be the ONE responsible for making key decisions.

Unfortunately, it was an argument the two young men were unable to settle and clashing egos would ultimately end the relatively short, 6-year run where the Beatles were, as John liked to say: "*the toppermost of the poppermost.*"[1]

When John installed a hanging bed at the Abbey Road recording studios so Yoko could observe – and comment on – all sessions, that's when Paul said: "I quit." So: *I, Me, Mine, was recorded without Paul.*[2] Decades later, when the biggest stars in the music business (from Michael Jackson to Diana Ross to Bruce Springsteen to Stevie Wonder) all gathered to record "We are the World," the equally famous producer of that recording session, Quincy Jones, hung a sign outside the studio that advised the famous participants to: "Leave your ego at the door."

In an article from Psychology Today, Mark Leary, Ph.D., explains: "terms that include 'ego' involve processes or reactions in which I, me, or mine figure prominently." When we say things like: I hate this or I dislike that, or even when a young child grabs a toy from her sibling and says: "That's mine!" That's the ego talking. Mindfulness teaches us how to recognize that demanding voice, and by so doing, we can separate what we truly need from what the ego THINKS it needs. *The true you is often willing to compromise where the EGO isn't.*

Think of three times where your ego (I, ME, MINE) played a destructive role in your life.

1. ______________________________
2. ______________________________
3. ______________________________

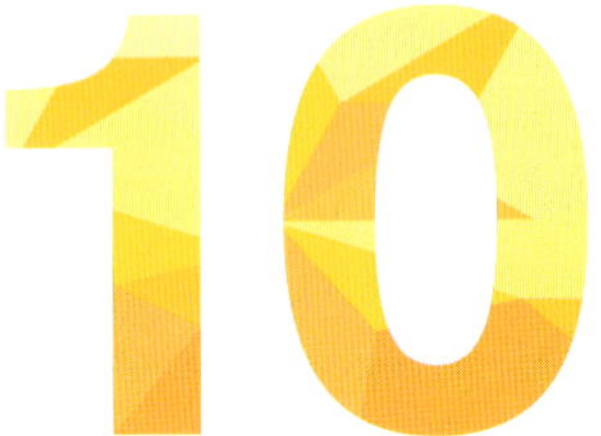

10. No-Self

According to mindfulness philosophy, the "self" is a mind-made construct that really doesn't exist. This is an extraordinary statement, which, at first look, seems to defy explanation. But it DOESN'T mean YOU don't exist. It simply means, this thing you MISTAKE for who you are (the self, or ego) which includes all your likes, dislikes, preferences, interpretations, memories, etcetera, is more or less just a software program YOU have installed in your own brain.

The Greek philosopher Epictetus famously said: "We are not bothered by events and circumstances *but by the views we take of them.*" This would suggest there's a defect in our "software" (in other words, our perception) that doesn't allow us to see things as they truly are.

While that may be true, mindfulness philosophy likes to take this idea *one step further.* That the real you is NOT your thoughts, your faulty beliefs or your perception. The real you *is the awareness below your thoughts and beliefs and perception.*

Once you embrace this concept of no-self (or, if you prefer, the awareness residing below the level of perception) there's real freedom in it. Think about how polarized we've all become lately and how people's opinions just seem so intractable. Everyone believes *their* software program (what THEY believe) is the only correct view, because we ALL mistake our thinking mind, for who we really are.

Remember when you were a kid and for a moment, when you first woke up, you'd forget it was Christmas or your birthday or some major holiday? A few seconds later, you'd remember what day it was, and you would be delighted! In these first waking moments, you briefly experience a kind of blank slate, just prior to the software program booting up.

Early one morning about five years ago, I woke up on the floor of a hotel room in Boston. For about thirty seconds I had no idea what I was doing on the floor in this strange room. (No, I wasn't out drinking the night before.) I remember feeling totally rested and relaxed, but I had no idea where I was, or why I had been sleeping on a mattress on the floor.

As I looked around, I saw my wife sleeping on a bed across the room and that's when my software program finally kicked in. We had gotten into a *huge* argument the night before. I said I would sleep on the sofa-bed, but the bar underneath the mattress was digging into my back, so I finally moved the mattress onto the floor and slept there the rest of the night.

It had been a bad argument and I said some things I now regretted. A moment prior to that, I was perfectly happy (no software program). Now I was perfectly miserable (program installed). I wondered; How could I get back to where I was the moment before? How could I reinvent myself moving forward? The answer was clear. I needed to apologize.

Up until that moment, I had mistaken that software program (or what we think of as "the self") for a kind of unalterable version of *who I was*. After that moment, I realized there was a me (what mindfulness refers to as "no-self") that was separate from the software program that could choose a whole new path.

This concept of no-self is one of the central tenets of mindfulness and yet it is seldom talked about in self-help books like this, because it's so complicated to explain. I hope I did a good job of explaining it to you. I personally didn't buy into this concept at *all* when I first read about it. Now, after my experience in Boston, I see how this concept operates in my life and in the lives of others. If you don't buy it, write three reasons why: If you do buy into it, think of three ways this understanding might help you in the future.

1. ______________________________
2. ______________________________
3. ______________________________

Ego Defined

Probably the best definition of ego I've ever heard is revealed in this story about a high-level government official who pays a visit to a Zen monk:

At the monastery the government official asks the monk a simple question: "What is Ego?"

The Zen monk quickly replies: "That's a stupid question."

Horrified by the monk's answer, the high-level governmental official indignantly shouts back: "Do you realize who you are talking to? I could make life very difficult for you."

To which the monk calmly responds: "That's ego."

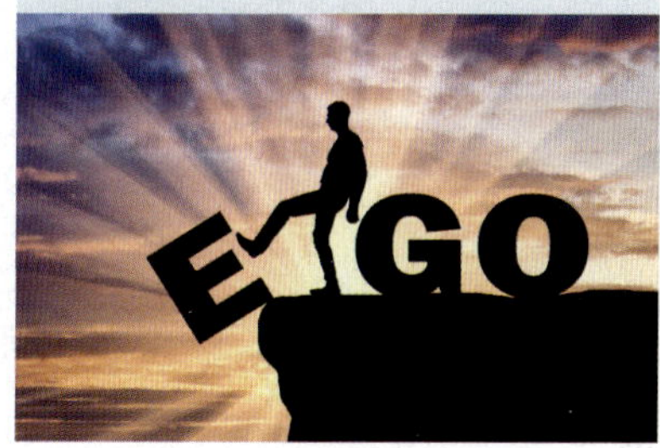

Chapter 5

Mindfulness at Work

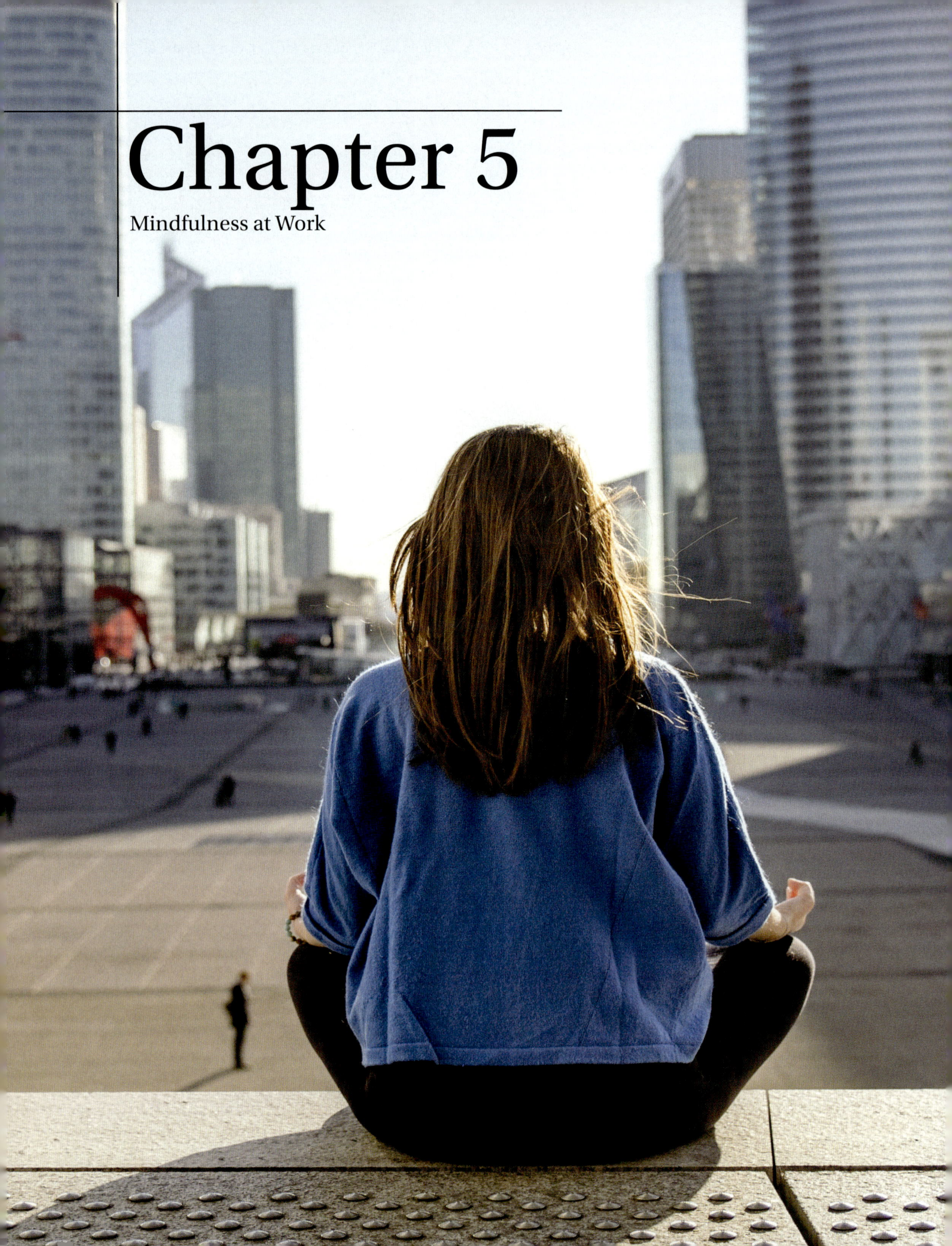

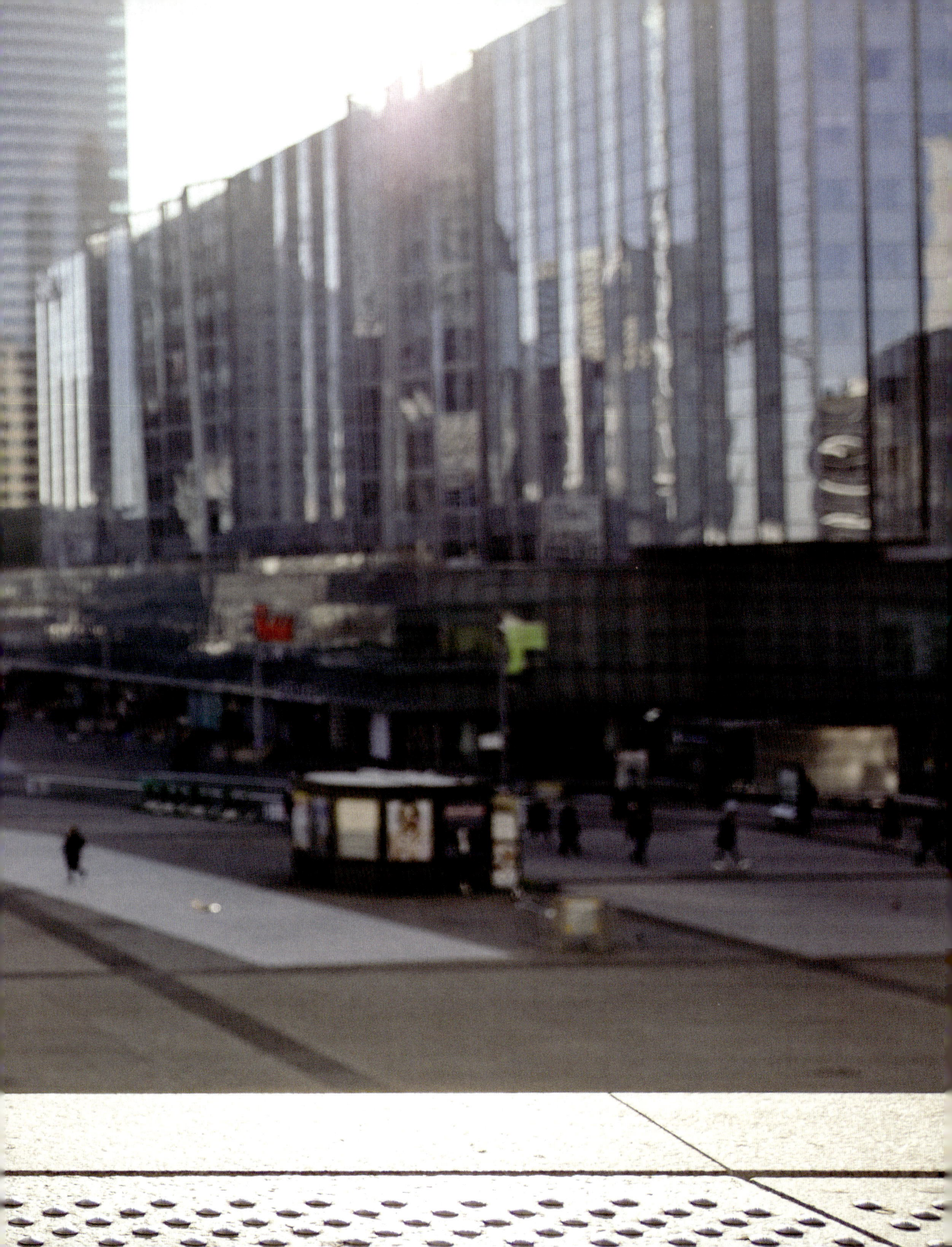

Chapter 5
Mindfulness at Work

Mark Bertolini was a rising star at the Aetna Insurance Company when he skied into a tree and fell down a thirty-foot ravine. By the time the ambulance got him to the Hospital, a priest was waiting to administer last rights. Nerves were severed in his shoulder and arm and numerous vertebrae in his neck were broken. Three surgeries, lots of rehab and lots of painkillers later he still had almost no use of his left arm and he was in constant pain.

That's when he turned to yoga and mindfulness for help. Eventually, Bertolini was back climbing the corporate ladder and, in 2010 he was named CEO of Aetna. Not only did Bertolini's star rise during his ascendency, so did the fortunes of his company, with its stock tripling in value while he was CEO. Bertolini attributes his amazing comeback and much of his personal success to yoga and mindfulness.

As CEO, he decided to share what he had learned about yoga and mindfulness with the entire organization. Employees could take these classes on company time. Any middle level manager who objected, got a personal note from Mark. Even Aetna's Chief Medical Officer had reservations at first, but Bertolini persisted, promising to track the results of the mindfulness and yoga classes on the workers who participated.

According to the New York Times: "More than one-quarter of the company's work force of 50,000 participated in at least one class, and those who did, reported on average, a 28 percent reduction in their stress levels, a 20 percent improvement in sleep quality and a 19 percent reduction in pain. They also were more effective on the job, gaining an average of 62 minutes per week of productivity each, which Aetna estimates was worth $3,000 per employee per year."[1]

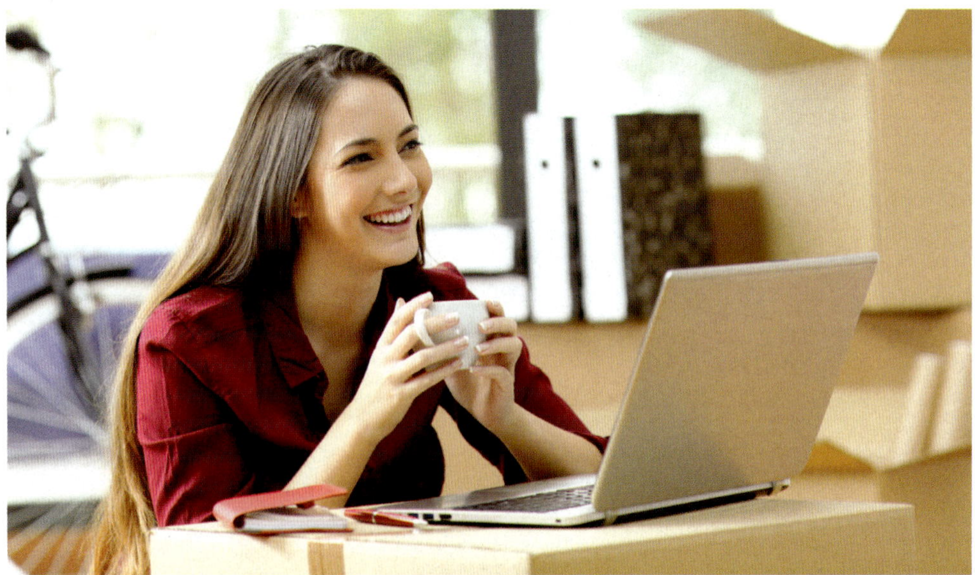

Another study done at Aetna, (in collaboration with researchers at Duke University) tracked the benefits of mindfulness in a randomized study of 239 employees. These volunteers were separated into two groups plus one control group that didn't get mindfulness or yoga training. The results of the study were published in the Journal of Occupational Medicine. "Compared with the control group, the mind-body interventions showed significantly greater improvements on perceived stress, sleep quality, and heart rate variability (a way to measure stress and anxiety)."[2]

At other organizations, like Google and Green Mountain Coffee, mindfulness is being rolled out to employees from the top down, by high level executives, who have caught the mindfulness bug and want to share it with employees at every level. But what do you do if your organization isn't offering free yoga and meditation classes? How do you introduce mindfulness into a workplace that isn't supporting it from the top down? Why not bring your understanding of mindfulness – if not your actual practice – to the workplace and share what you know with others.

That's exactly, what a self-described "closet meditator," Janice Marturano, did at General Mills. She started teaching others what she knew about meditation and mindfulness. Gradually her love of mindfulness caught on at General Mills and turned into a groundswell of interest. Now, there are dedicated meditation rooms scattered throughout the entire organization and mindfulness meditation is practiced at all levels of the company.[3]

Here's how to bring your mindfulness practice to work, just like Janice Marturano. Pick your favorite exercise from chapter 2 and give yourself a little 2-minute break whenever you are feeling frazzled or distracted. Concepts from Chapter 4 like impermanence, non-attachment, name it and tame it or asking yourself the question: How am I doing right now? all come in handy in the workplace.

Don't forget, the meditation practice you have at home is going to come in handy at work, too. Here's why: Every time you meditate (at home) you are strengthening neural pathways between your prefrontal cortex (the control center of the brain) and the mid-brain (the emotional center of the brain) where the amygdala is located and where the stress response begins.

As the result of your daily practice, not only are you going to feel less stressed, you'll be able to control your stress response, while your stress is happening. This is a huge advantage in the workplace. You'll be better able to concentrate, turn off distractions, think more clearly, handle difficult emotions, and communicate better, too. You will be more able to remain calm in challenging situations, you'll most likely sleep better, and as the result of ALL these benefits put together: *you'll be more productive at work.*[4]

In other words, your at-home meditation practice, will follow you to work every day. Eventually people will start asking you: "How do you remain so "Zen" all the time? If you think they are ready to hear the real answer, start sharing it with them. In that way your practice will grow and influence others who may want to try it too.

On the mindfulness retreat I participated in, which was specifically designed for business leaders, Jon Kabat-Zinn summed up the workplace benefits of mindfulness in this way: "Mindfulness increases your personal power. Your power isn't siphoned off by the need to be right. It isn't sucked up by yesterday's argument and it isn't challenged by tomorrow's fear. Being here right now restores your power, frees you from old arguments and liberates you from fear."

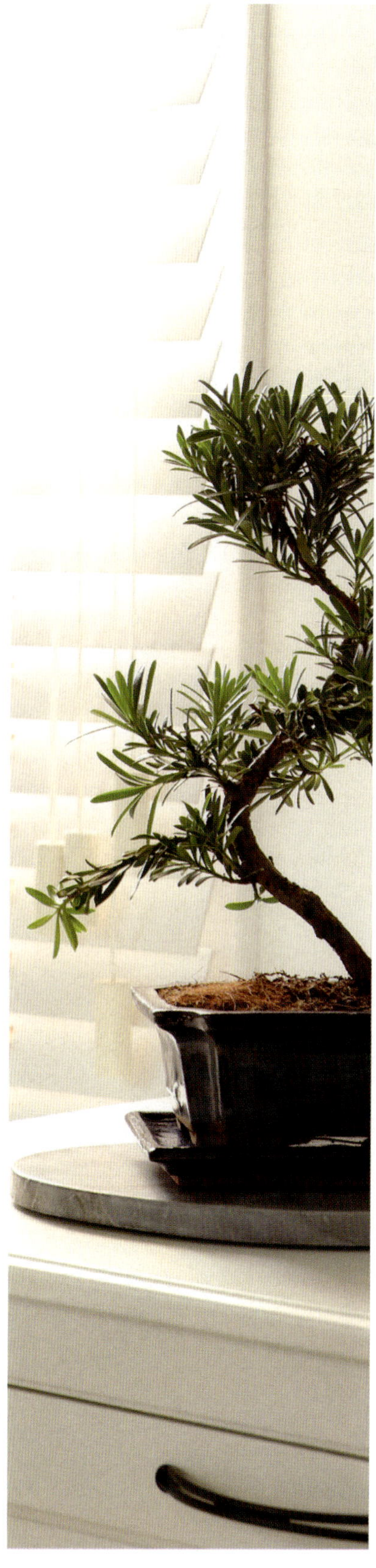

Myth of Multi-tasking

Mindfulness and multi-tasking don't really mix. Study after study has shown that multi-tasking, is, in fact, less efficient than mindfully tackling one task at a time. This occurs for several reasons. **1.** We are more likely to make mistakes when we multi-task and **2.** Each time we switch from one activity to another it takes several minutes before we really lock our attention in on the new task.

Most people don't realize that our attention span only goes so far. When we multi-task, we are not increasing our attention, but dividing it up into smaller buckets. Let's say you are attending the morning sales meeting at work and to that meeting you've brought an egg sandwich, coffee, and your laptop. You are all set to multi-task. Since the meeting doesn't have much to do with you today, you decide to work on a report that's due on your boss's desk by noon.

Continued on page 43.

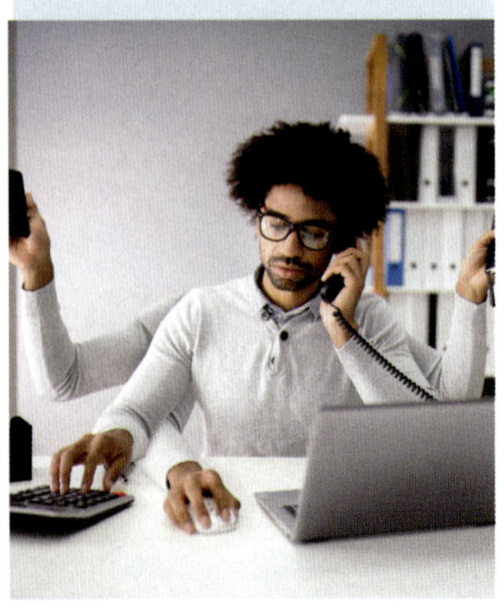

"Being in the moment is about what's happening right now," he went on to say. "And every moment is different from the one that just preceded it. So, if something or someone bugged you yesterday, and it's still bothering you today, chances are you're grasping on to an old story."[5]

Maybe the story you are grasping onto is: *My workplace is unfair; I have the world's worst boss; I'll never succeed in this place; Nobody likes me; Or, my coworkers are of no use at all.* In mindfulness, this tendency to make overly-generalized statements is sometimes referred to as having a "narrative view" of life.

When you have a narrative view, if someone says something unkind one day, and is perfectly nice to you the next, but you are still holding onto what happened the day before, that's a *narrative* view. A moment by moment view, as John Kabat-Zinn says, will give you your power back. You will operate in a productive bubble called the NOW. The now is where the action is. It's where your life is going on.

Being in the moment gives you a competitive edge. You don't let little things bother you, because 1. You've rewired your brain to *not let little things bother you* (aka, trait changes) and 2. You know (better than anyone else in the office) that in another moment this little annoying thing will be reduced to a memory trace and you will be focused on a whole different moment. And when big things happen that DO need to be addressed, you will address them calmly and in *that* moment.

Mark Bertolini and Trish Meili (The Central Park Jogger) could have never recovered from their traumatic injuries without taking this moment-by-moment view and letting go of the narrative view. When we take the present moment view, we let go of old hurts, forgive ourselves for our mistakes, we forgive others for their mistakes and *move on.* The only thing you can do anything about is whatever might be happening in this moment.

As you consider how to be more mindful at work, think about taking full advantage of opportunities throughout your day to tune into the present moment:

Start each day mindfully. When you first sit down at your desk or workstation, take a moment to check in with your own body. Notice where it is touching the chair, where your feet touch the floor, where your skin is exposed to the air. Take a deep breath in and a deep breath out.

Take mindfulness breaks. Find a quiet spot – or moment – where you can just listen to the sounds in the room. Do a short meditation on these sounds or notice your breathing for just two minutes.

Create a mindful lunch. Go for a walk outside. Have your lunch in a nearby park or under a tree. Think about what you are eating while you are eating. Savor every bite.

Be mindful on your commute to work. Aim to arrive early, so you don't spend the entire time worrying about whether you are going to be late. Take public transportation, ride a bike or if you must drive, see if you can take back roads that aren't so heavily clogged with traffic. Every choice you make about your route to work, or your mode of transportation, should be made thoughtfully, knowing that these choices will lead to greater peace of mind throughout your day.

Try single-tasking. If you can, set aside 60 to 90 minutes each day to work on one project, without interruption. The more you focus on completing just one task, the more it will seem like a mindfulness meditation.

Work from home. If it's available to you, try working from home in a place where you can do it without family members interrupting your workflow. Your entire day will be more mindful.

Find tasks that encourage "flow." Any tasks that are challenging enough to require your full attention hold the promise of putting you into a *flow state*, where you feel relaxed and even rejuvenated, *while you work.* Sometimes you will need to leave your comfort zone, just a bit, in order to find the right level of challenge where your attention is captivated enough to achieve flow. Volunteer to do jobs that take you into new territory, and this sense of flow may soon follow.

Take a few minutes to meditate when you get home from work. Take five minutes alone, in your room, before you start interacting with your roommates, friends or family members. Build some mindfully created space or boundaries between work and home.

Consider taking your shower when you come home from work, rather than in the morning when you are feeling rushed. This way, your shower can become a totally relaxing experience where you take your time and think about what you are doing while you are doing it.

Work out or meditate in the morning before leaving for work. Being mindful is often an inside out affair. When your body feels good you feel good. When you feel good, you can concentrate better, focus more easily, and ultimately be more mindful.

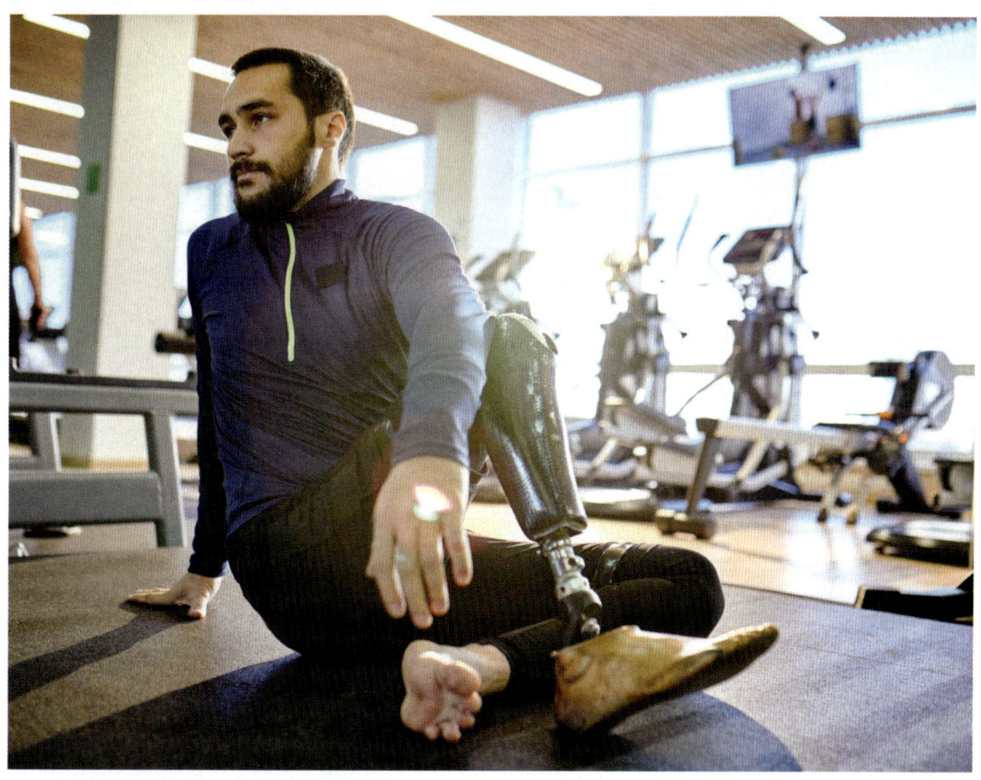

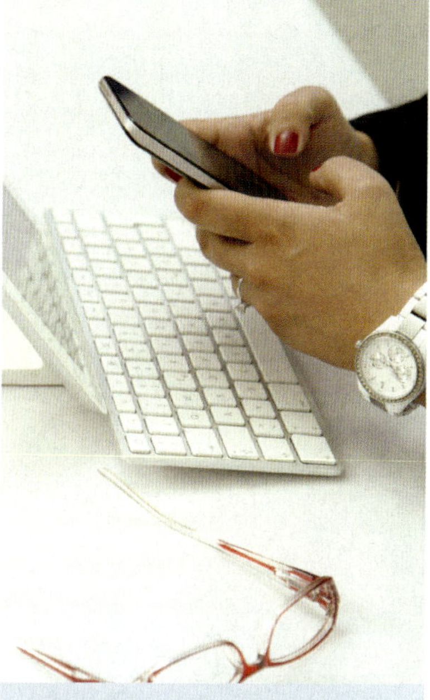

Myth of Multi-tasking

Most of your attention – let's say 60 percent - is focused on the report. But there's also a part of you, let's say 30%, that's paying attention to the meeting, to make sure there's nothing being said that applies to you. The other 10 percent of your attention is split between sips of coffee and bites of your sandwich. With this subdivided attention, you are MUCH more likely to spill your coffee, drip grease on your shirt, or make a mistake on that report.

Make just one misstep, and ALL the efficiency you thought you were gaining, is lost and then some. To top it off, as the result of multi-tasking (and making an inevitable mistake), you may feel frazzled and stressed. (And not really enjoy the egg sandwich or the coffee.)

Chapter 6

Calm Down: Using Meditation to Self-regulate Your Nervous System

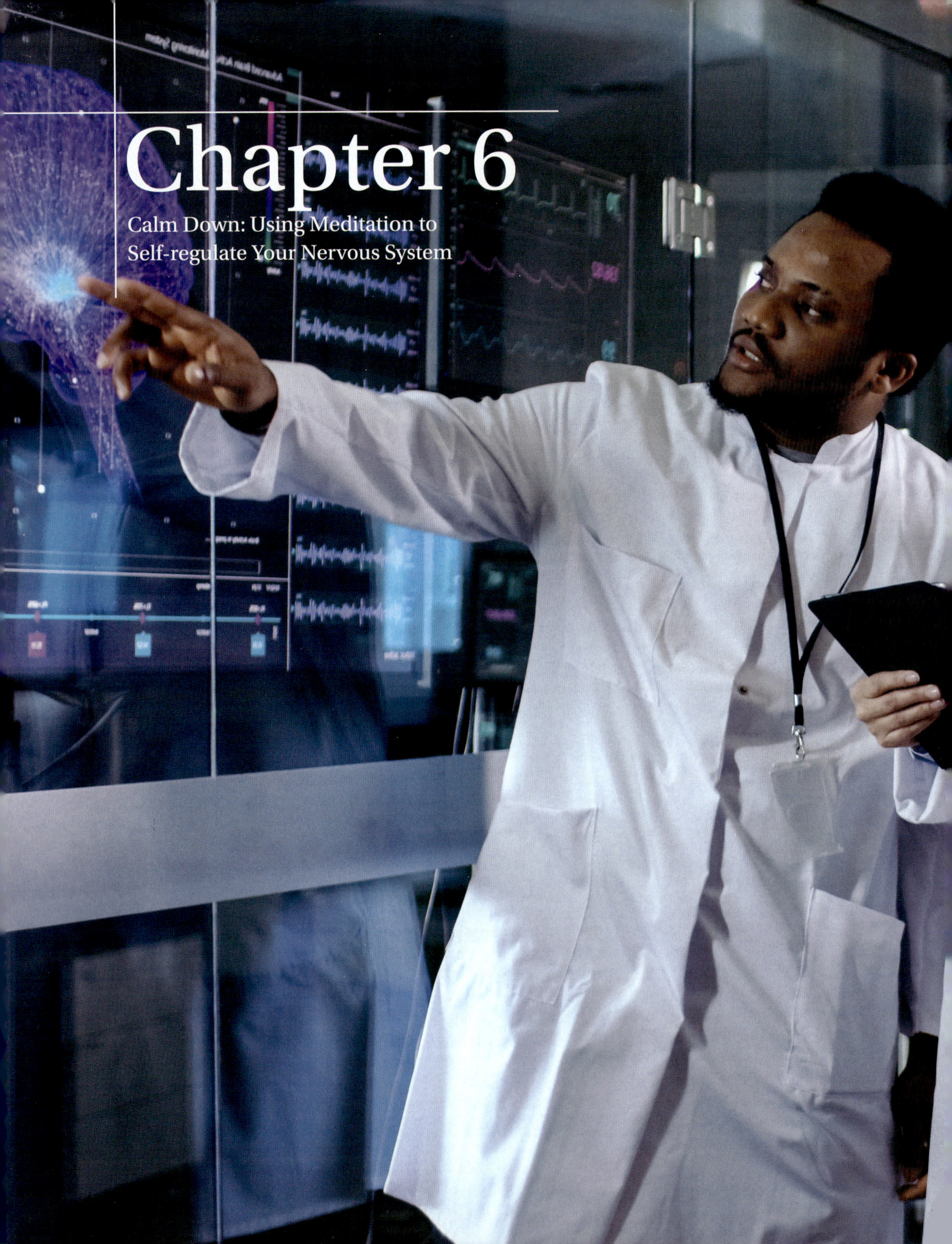

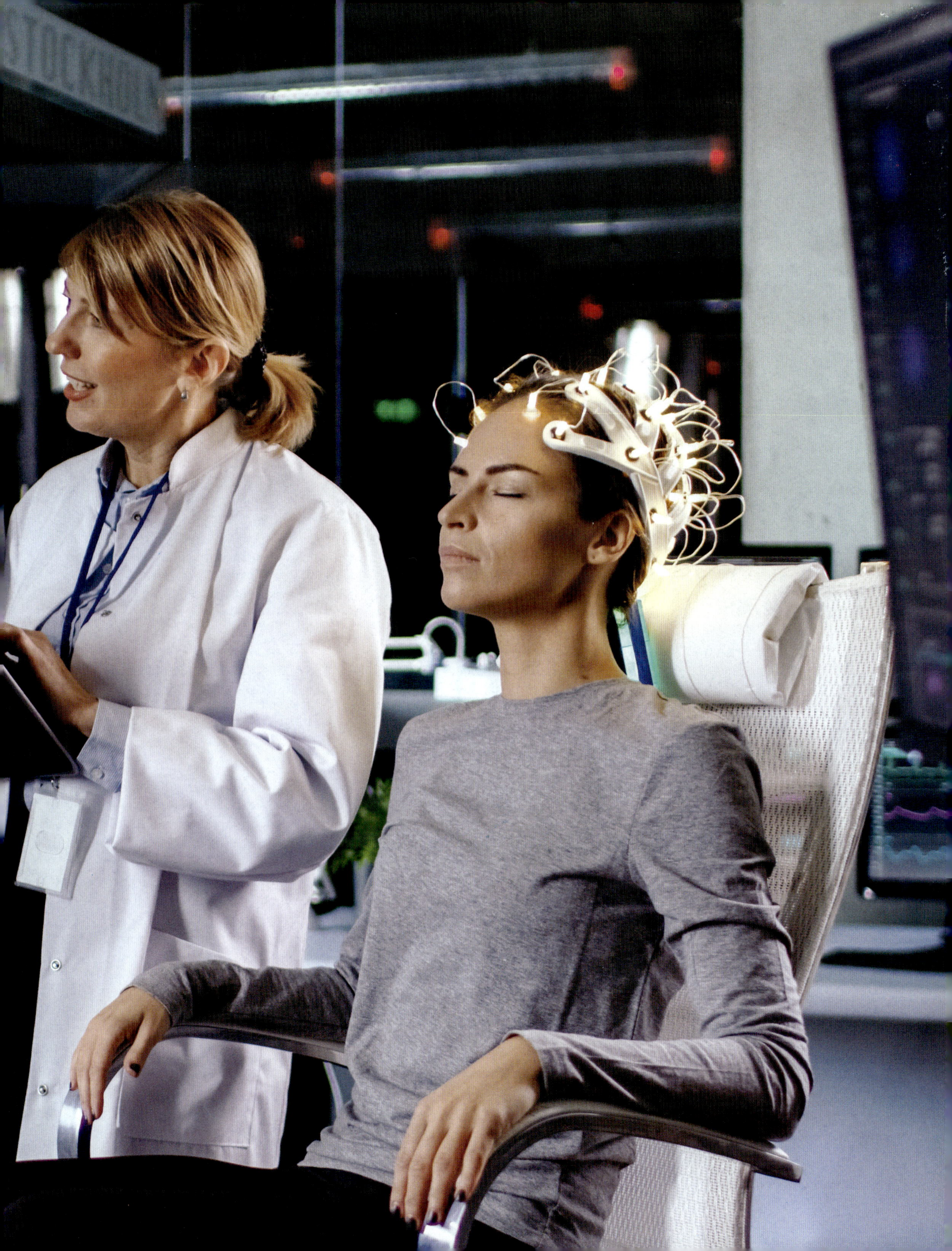

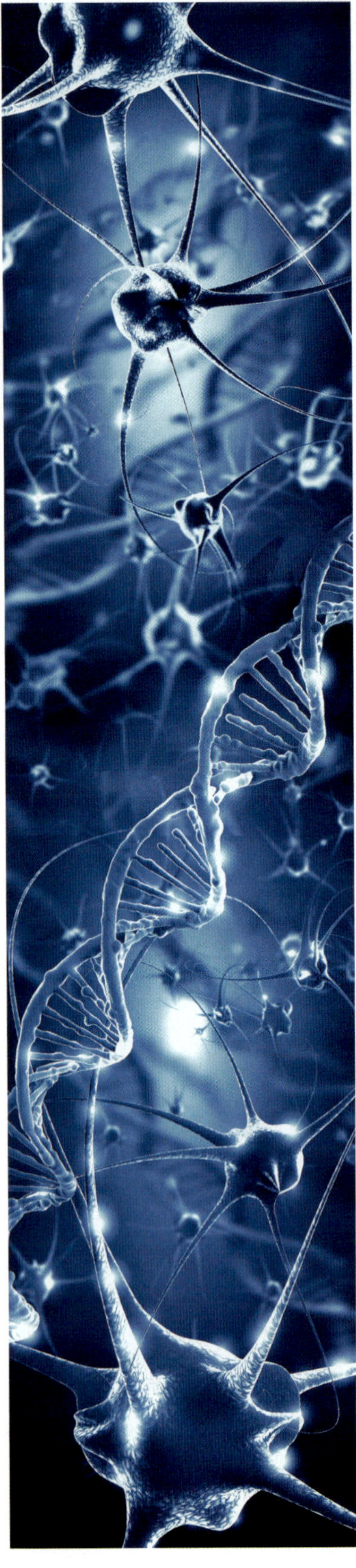

Chapter 6
Calm Down: Using Meditation to Self-regulate Your Nervous System

In the early 1970s, Herbert Benson, M.D., a professor at Harvard University, was approached by a group of students he described as "hippies," who asked him if he could monitor their vital functions while meditating. At that time, Benson was working in the same lab at Harvard where, fifty years earlier, Walter B. Cannon had discovered and named the *fight or flight* response. Cannon's work studying stress would make him world famous. Benson's work studying relaxation would make him world famous, too.

One of the students told Benson he thought he could self-regulate his nervous system simply by meditating. Up until that point, Western science held that the *autonomic* nervous system couldn't be controlled voluntarily. It ran on autopilot, with no conscious control exercised by the individual. Yet these meditators were pretty sure they could control autonomic functions like heart rate, breathing rate, skin temperature and blood pressure. If Benson could hook them up to his biofeedback equipment that might provide the scientific evidence needed to elevate meditation beyond what the Western world thought of it at the time: A passing fad, *with no real therapeutic value.*

Benson agreed, but under one condition. The students would have to come by his lab at night, when no one would see what they were doing. Benson wasn't worried about his colleagues stealing his research, he was worried about losing his job.[1] He thought the university wouldn't look too kindly on the idea of one of their brightest scientists studying something as *frivolous* as meditation.

But Benson knew his students were right about one thing. If they could do what they thought they could do, simply by meditating, his machines would prove it. *And that would be big news.* In his research, he had come across reports of monks, swamis and gurus in India who claimed they could do similar feats of autonomic control using nothing but their own (unique) meditative practices.

There were swamis who claimed they could be buried alive for hours in an airtight box by slowing down their metabolism. There were gurus who said they could stop their hearts; there were monks who said they could raise their skin temperature in specific places on their body. Benson would eventually go and study some of these unusual people in India, but for now, there was no solid proof that anybody had ANY control over their autonomic nervous system. And studying his students, right in his own back yard to see if there was any validity to these claims, was way cheaper than traveling to India.

Once Benson hooked these meditators up to his biofeedback devices, he could see clearly that they could voluntarily control *involuntary* functions. They could raise and lower their heart rates, increase their skin temperature and, on occasion, lower their blood pressure, using nothing more than meditation techniques to do it. By studying this and writing about it, Benson sold millions and millions of copies of his classic book, THE RELAXATION RESPONSE.[2]

The particular style of meditation that the students used was called (and still is called) Transcendental Meditation or TM. TM is more or less a "brand" of meditation which can cost a lot of money (as much as $1,000) to learn from a yoga guru or certified instructor. In TM, you are assigned a special mantra (a Sanskrit word or phrase) that is chosen just for you, by the guru or instructor. "Om Shanti" would be an example of a popular mantra assigned by a guru.

After attending a lecture in London in 1967, conducted by the founder of TM, Maharishi Mahesh Yogi, John, Paul, George and Ringo (AKA, The Beatles) flew off to India, to spend several weeks studying meditation at the guru's ashram in Rishikesh, India. That helped put meditation – and in particular, TM - on the map. Paul McCartney and Ringo Starr still practice TM to this day. And now there are lots of famous TM practitioners including Jerry Seinfeld, Katy Perry, Lena Dunham, and Jennifer Aniston, to name just a few. Many of these stars talk openly about how meditation has changed their lives.[3]

Just before he died, the Maharishi decided to raise the price of learning TM to the high level that it is today. His theory was, that if only famous people and influencers could afford it that would spread the word about the benefits of TM even faster.

But as Benson studied his own students more and more, he realized that the important benefits of meditation could easily be derived *without* taking an expensive course. His research confirmed that almost any comforting word or phrase could be substituted for a mantra and work just as well. In his book, Benson suggests other possible "mantras" including the words *peace* or *one* or even a short phrase like *I am feeling more and more relaxed.*

In terms of popular psychology, whatever word or phrase you have chosen to say, quickly becomes an "operant conditioner" and just repeating it, along with regular practice, will eventually trigger the body to go into a relaxed state. (Just like the sound of a bell would automatically cause Pavlov's dogs to salivate.)

When he first started exploring words and phrases that might substitute for a mantra, Benson asked his students to try counting slowing from one to ten, over and over. This turned out to be problematic because, while meditating, his students would often lose track of where they were in the count and get frustrated. He thought it was enormously funny that, at least while meditating, his Harvard students *couldn't even count to ten!*[4] But this inability to keep track of the count, pointed out a potential snag in any style of

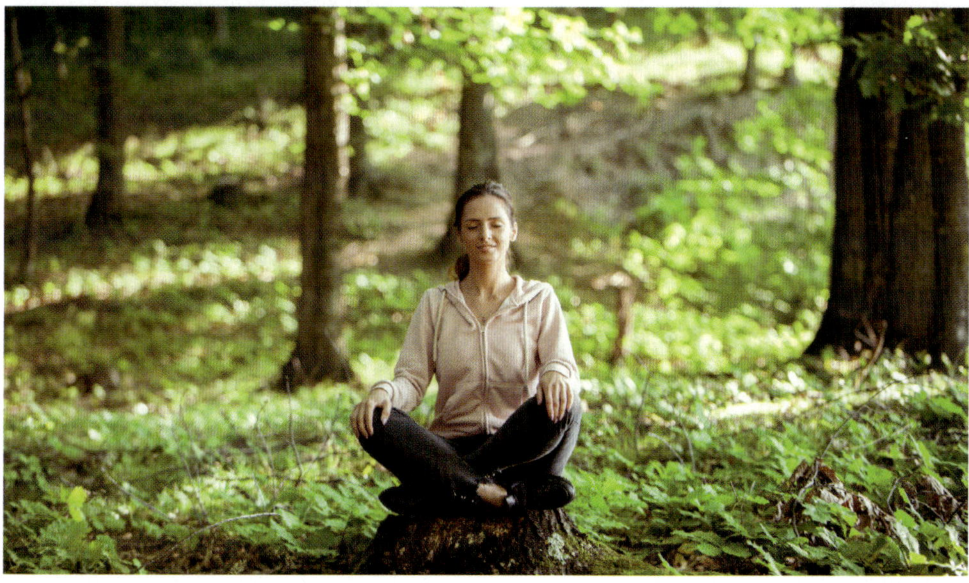

An Amygdala Hijacking

The stress response begins in the amygdala, a small almond-shaped area in the middle part of the brain. Whenever the amygdala senses a threat, it sends a signal to the prefrontal cortex, (PFC) which is responsible for interpreting the level of that threat and its validity. But if the threat seems urgent enough, the amygdala doesn't wait for an interpretation. It simply hijacks the PFC, even in cases where the threat is a false alarm.

Let me give you an example: My first car would occasionally backfire which sounded like a gunshot going off nearby. As a result, I would reflexively duck for cover. My reaction happened instantly and without me thinking about it. A few seconds later, my PFC would reinterpret the data and say: No real threat; just the car backfiring. That's a short-lived amygdala hijacking ending in a false alarm.

When the danger is perceived to be real, the amygdala exerts certain controls over the brain and the body. It makes you pay attention to the threat, and if you are unable to remove it, the amygdala is going to make you feel anxious until you do. If you've ever had trouble trying to "think straight" when you're in the middle of a crisis situation, now you know why.

The good news is, meditation helps us to control the amygdala, even in situations like this. By strengthening the neural connections between the PFC and the amygdala, long-term meditators learn to self-regulate this unwanted amygdala reactivity.

meditation: *Mind wandering.* This is one of the key issues that all beginning meditators struggle with. Mostly it is addressed in all styles of meditation with the same simple advice: If your mind wanders, without judgement, (such as: "I can't believe my mind wandered again." Or, "I'm terrible at this") simply bring it back to whatever it is you are focusing on, whether that's a mantra, a pleasing word or phrase, your breathing, or the sound of the rain on the roof. Mind-wandering is just part of the process.

In his book the Relaxation Response, which was the first popular book to really lay out and prove the therapeutic value of meditation, Benson describes his four ground rules for learning how to meditate.[5] In order to meditate, you need:

1. **A quiet environment.** Find a quiet place where you won't be disturbed.
2. **An object to dwell on.** Repeat a calming word or phrase silently to yourself.
3. **A passive attitude.** You can't force yourself into a meditative state. (So, if your mind wanders, gently bring it back to the word or phrase you have chosen to meditate on.)
4. **A comfortable position.** (Sitting in a chair, back straight, hands on your lap, feet flat on the floor or sitting on a pillow on the floor with your legs crossed.)

This was Benson's own version of TM, sometimes referred to as concentration meditation, where the main goal is to concentrate or meditate on a mantra or as Benson provided, a calming word or phrase. Mindfulness meditation, which needs no mantra, and costs nothing to learn, simply requires you to focus on anything that brings you into the present moment. It is often referred to as insight meditation or sometimes "vipassana meditation."

Both styles of meditation, as Benson's research would show, allow a person to maintain conscious control over his or her own nervous system. As Benson explains in his book, this has some very interesting benefits including peace of mind, improved focus and reduced stress. Since it's the polar opposite of Walter Cannon's fight or flight response, Benson logically named this new answer to stress: *The Relaxation Response.*

Long before Benson wrote the Relaxation Response, western scientists already knew that the nervous system was divided into two branches, the sympathetic and the parasympathetic. These two branches travel throughout the body on the back of one very long nerve called the vagus nerve. Like the word vagabond, which is a person that travels from place to place, the vagus nerve travels from place to place throughout the body. Physicians before 1900 were fascinated and equally mystified by this one nerve, which snaked through the entire body and made contact with all the major organs and muscles.

Why would one neural highway need to connect with so many different organs these early scientists wondered? Up until this point in the history of medicine, it was thought that, while all these major organs and muscles were connected to and controlled by the brain, they still operated independently of each other. Why would one nerve connect in all these different places?

After Walter Cannon came along and discovered the fight or flight response, the purpose of the vagus nerve became clear. It was designed to muster up the help of every organ and muscle in the entire body in one unified, instantaneous response to an immediate threat. The fight or flight response and the stress response are terms – that not quite accurately – are often used interchangeably.

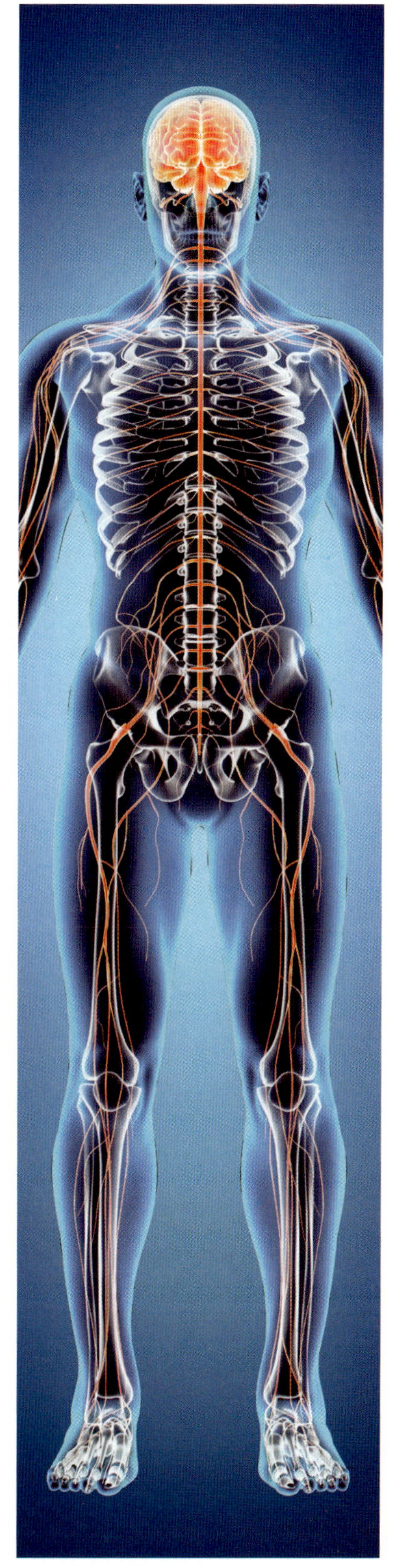

The *sympathetic* nervous system (delivered by the vagus nerve) prepares the body to fight or flee. The *parasympathetic* nervous system (also delivered by the vagus nerve) tells the body when it's time to slow down and rest (aka, rest and digest). When someone or something appears threatening, and you feel your muscles tense, that's the *sympathetic* nervous system being activated. When you yawn, and you start feeling tired, that's the *parasympathetic* nervous system being activated.

When one part of the system is turned on, the other part is turned off. Benson's work proved that, not only meditation, but other activities like yoga, deep breathing, and progressive muscle relaxation could turn the sympathetic nervous system (fight or flight) off and the parasympathetic nervous system (rest and digest) on.

One morning long ago, I remember the office manager buzzing me on the intercom at my first job and telling me Marlon Brando was on the line.

"You're kidding."

"No, the guy on the phone says he's Marlon Brando."

Figuring it was just a prank call I picked up the phone. "Hello?" I asked, waiting for some random teenager to pull some practical joke.

"This is Marlon Brando. I understand you have a film in your library with Dr. Elmer Green on Biofeedback."

"Yes, that's true, I said," knowing by the sound of his unmistakable voice, that I really was talking to the THE Godfather, a man whose voice, *I had imitated*, occasionally uttering lines in conversation like "*I could have been a contender,*" and "*I'm gonna make him an offer he can't refuse.*"

"How can I help you?" I said, trying to sound business-like but pinching myself to make sure I wasn't dreaming.

"I recently spoke to Dr. Green at the Menninger Foundation, about treating my migraine headaches with biofeedback. He thought that seeing your film might be of some help."

My boss, Elda Hartley, had created this film, just before I started working there. She and Dr. Green had traveled around India together in search of the same swamis and gurus who could control involuntary functions of the body. In other words, they were looking for people who could self-regulate their nervous systems.

The resulting film focused primarily on the use of biofeedback for treating migraine headaches. They weren't able to meet with anyone in India who had these extraordinary powers, so most of the film was shot at the Menninger Foundation Clinic in Topeka, Kansas. That's where Dr. Green was teaching groups of people how to control their migraine headaches - without medication – by just using biofeedback. It was Dr. Green's pioneering work in the 1970's that launched thousands of biofeedback clinics throughout this country in the decade or so that followed. Marlon Brando wanted to hear about this new information from the source: Dr. Green himself.

I made the arrangements to send a copy of the film to Brando's home in Malibu.

A couple of months later, Dr. Green visited our office in Connecticut. Like Marlon Brando, I was eager to learn about biofeedback from the man who had practically invented it.[6] "Biofeedback," he explained, "simply monitors internal states, it doesn't change those internal states one bit." He defined it as the feedback of internal (biological) information that we don't normally have access to.

"I teach people various techniques like visualization, deep breathing, progressive muscle relaxation, guided imagery and so forth, and that's what changes the internal states. The biofeedback equipment simply monitors those states and shows the person what progress they are making."

Back at his lab in Kansas which I visited sometime later, Dr. Green had all kinds of sophisticated equipment that could measure heart rate, skin temperature, perspiration, blood pressure, breathing rate and one machine that could measure brainwaves called an electroencephalograph, or EEG machine. Dr. Green used that machine to measure meditation states. What Dr. Green and others discovered, was the more relaxed a person became during meditation, the more their brainwaves would slow down.

Early researchers named these different brainwave states: Beta, Alpha, Theta and Delta. At 14 to 30 cycles per second or above, Beta brain waves predominate. This is considered to be normal waking consciousness. At 8 to 13 cycles per second Alpha waves predominate. These wave lengths usually occur in people who are meditating or sleeping lightly. Theta waves (4 to 7 cycles per second) are found in people who are sound asleep, and Delta waves, which occur below 3.5 cycles per second, are usually found only in people who are in a very deep sleep. People in Delta are virtually unconscious and very hard to wake up.

After the biofeedback film was made and long before my visit to the Clinic, a world-famous guru, Swami Rama, arrived at the Menninger Foundation to be studied. Dr. Green was excited to see what they would learn when they hooked Swami Rama up to their various biofeedback devices. The Swami did not disappoint. He promptly demonstrated that he could stop his heart, which he did, according to Dr. Green, for 17 seconds.[7] He also demonstrated that he could simultaneously raise the temperature in one spot on the palm of his hand 10-degrees warmer than another spot only an inch away. The Swami said this skill was more difficult than stopping his heart.[8]

Even though the Swami didn't know anything about brainwaves, he knew he had control over different mind states, which he could bring about voluntarily, on command, by meditating. Dr. Green wanted to hook him up to the EEG to see what brainwaves the Swami produced while meditating. This is an account of what happened written by Dr. Green himself:

> The Swami produced theta EEG rhythms at will in the occipital regions. This he called "Stilling the conscious and bringing forward the unconscious" a state he described as being "noisy" and unpleasant. When I asked him exactly what he meant by that he said: "All the things I wanted to do and didn't do, all the things other people wanted me to do that I didn't do, and all of the things I should have done but didn't do, came up and began screaming at me at the same time. It is not pleasant. Usually I keep it turned off, but sometimes it's good to see what is in there."[9]

Lucid Dreaming

When I first started meditating, I didn't know what lucid dreams were. I thought that when I had them, that was a sign that I was meditating. Now I know that while meditating, I sometimes momentarily fall into a light sleep and dream. Because it's only momentary and very light, I'm aware of it while it's happening. These dreams, are almost always delightful.

My best lucid dream ever came at a wellness conference. I was sitting in a circle, in a room with 20 other people. We had all been meditating with eyes closed for about 10 minutes. Suddenly I saw myself, flying above the room looking down at all the meditators. I was aware of what the instructor was actually saying at that moment: "OK everyone come back into the room and open your eyes."

I remember thinking: I've got to get back down in my chair. I can't be floating around up here above the room. When I opened up my eyes, I felt wonderful. It was almost as if I had had an "out of body experience." I've had many other lucid dreams since then while meditating but none were ever quite as vivid as that one.

The next day they asked the Swami if he could go even deeper into meditation. Again, he had no idea what delta brainwaves were, (the slowest brainwaves, usually only found in someone in a very deep sleep) but he did know he could get into a deeper state of relaxation, which he called Yogic Sleep. The Swami also promised he would demonstrate several more things for Dr. Green and his team while he was in that state of yogic sleep.

Just as the Swami pledged, he started producing Delta brainwaves on cue. But he also predicted that, when the session was over, he would remember everything that happened while he was in that state, and he would arouse himself, whenever Dr. Green requested, without need of a clock or any prompting whatsoever. He explained that, although it might look like he was sleeping, he assured them that he would be totally conscious the whole time and remember everything that happened while he was in that state.

The Swami laid down on a couch that was installed in the lab, and Dr. Green's team hooked him up to the EEG. They asked him to remain in this state, for 25 minutes. During the meditation, one of the members of Dr. Green's team remained in the room to check on the Swami and would quietly read a sentence she had written down to test the Swami's memory. The first sentence she read was: "Today the sun is shining but tomorrow it may rain."

While on the couch, Swami Rama appeared to be asleep and the observer reported that he was snoring lightly. Precisely at 25 minutes the Swami (who had no way of knowing the time) woke himself up, and a few minutes later, not only was able to precisely recall 3 out of the 4 sentences with total accuracy, (in the fourth one he got the gist of it) he also pointed out some unplanned, random noise that had occurred during that same time period. Dr. Green and his team were astounded, to say the least. [10]

With their combined research, Dr. Green and Dr. Benson were able to prove that meditators and swamis could self-regulate their own nervous systems: That they could achieve voluntary control over systems of the body that up until that point were considered involuntary; That they could take conscious control of their nervous systems to not only relax themselves, but potentially relieve chronic health problems like migraine headaches, hypertension and certain gastro-intestinal disorders.

It wasn't until Dr. Benson and Dr. Green came along that Western scientists fully understood that there was an off switch to this comprehensive alarm system, delivered throughout the body, by the vagus nerve. That the parasympathetic branch of this very same vagus nerve, could be consciously used to turn OFF the fight or flight response and activate what Benson named The Relaxation Response. These pioneering Western scientists both proved beyond a shadow of a doubt that when one part of the system is turned on, the other part of the system is turned off.

We also know beyond a shadow of a doubt, that frequently turning on this alarm system in situations where we can't fight and we can't flee, leads to all kinds of chronic health problems like back pain, neck pain, stomach pain, headaches, high blood pressure and heart disease.[11] So we absolutely need to have techniques in place, such as the ones you are learning about in this book, including mindfulness meditation, concentration meditation, deep breathing, progressive muscle relaxation and visualization, that can turn *on* the relaxation response and turn *off* the fight or flight response.

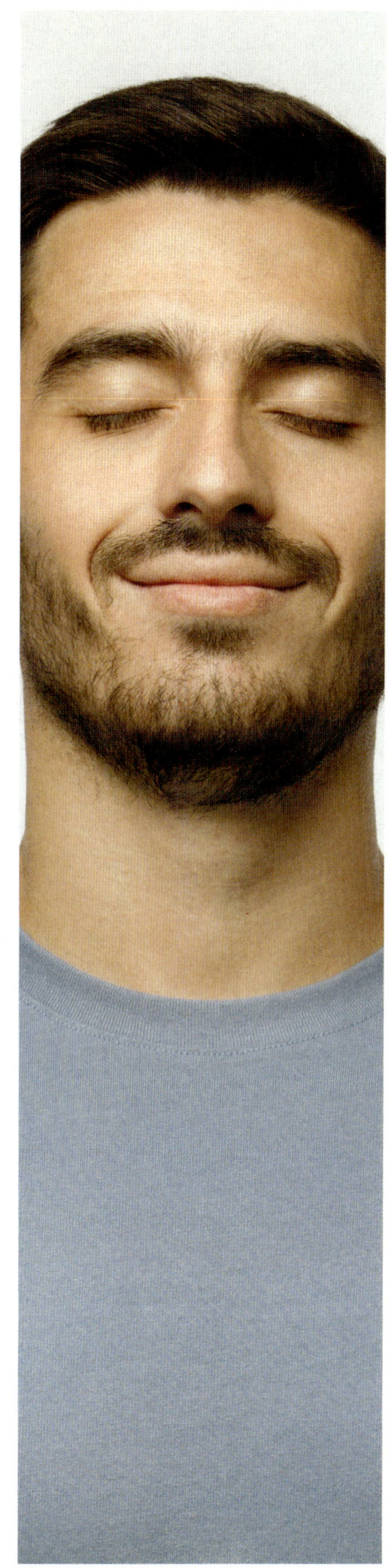

Chapter 7
Mindfulness as Integrative Medicine

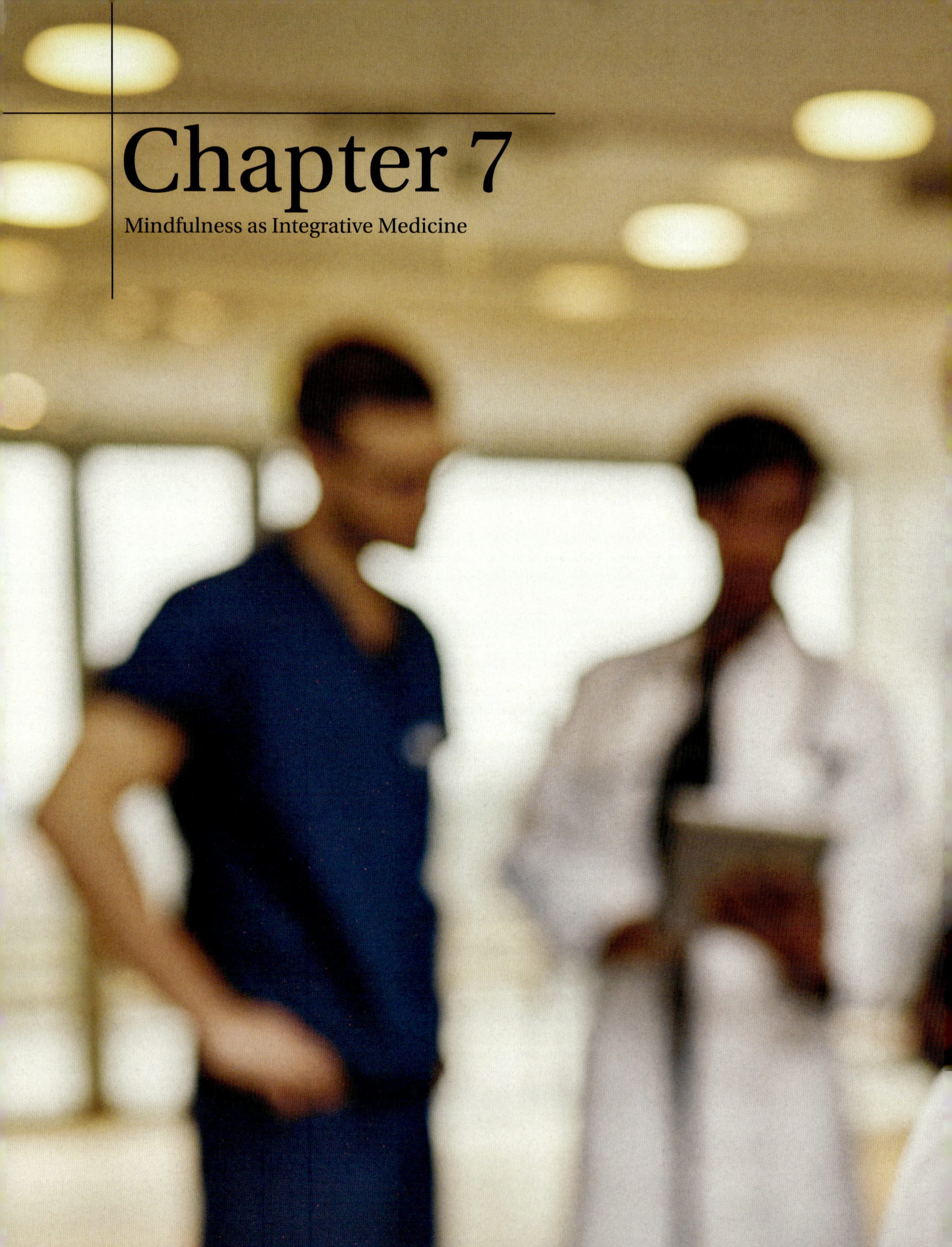

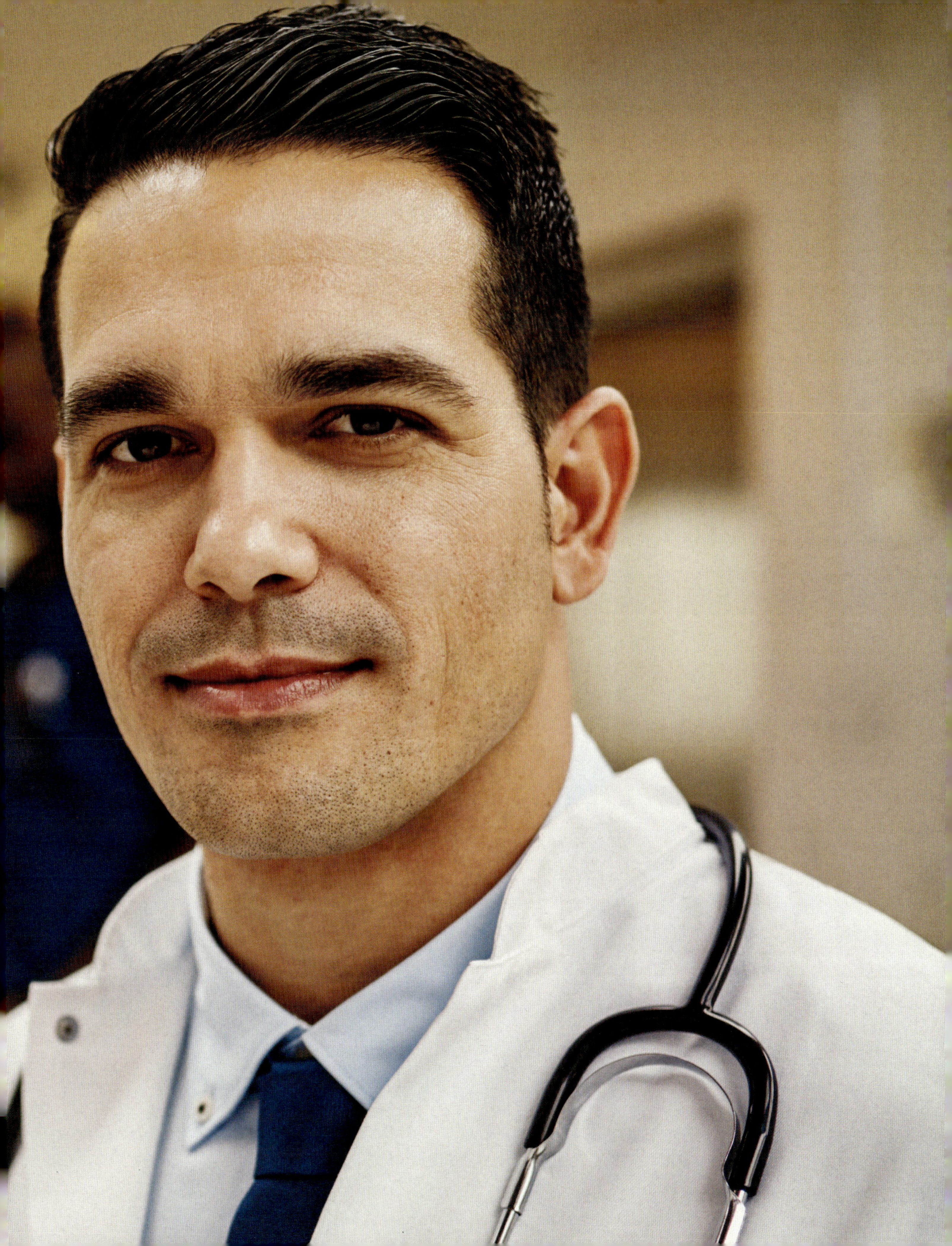

Chapter 7
Mindfulness as Integrative Medicine: First Do No Harm

When Jon Kabat-Zinn started his Mindfulness-based Stress Reduction Clinic at the University of Massachusetts Medical Center, at first, there was no mention of mindfulness at all. It was just The Stress Reduction and Relaxation Clinic. Initially, the doctors there didn't quite know what to make of this new clinic. But if there was a patient that nobody else could fix, the doctors would concede: "Why don't you try going to the Stress Reduction Clinic, they *might* be able to help you."

That's about when Jon Kabat-Zinn started telling his new arrivals: "*As long as you are still breathing, there is more right with you than what is wrong with you.*" Much to everyone's surprise, The Stress Reduction Clinic DID help these patients that nobody else could fix. And it's easy to see why. If stress is a primary driver of your dis-ease, you must lower that stress, in order to address the root of the problem.

You might have already noticed that your insomnia, your recurrent colds, your heart palpitations, your blue moods, your chronic pain, your migraines, your hives and perhaps even your more serious auto-immune disease symptoms, often flare-up ONLY during times of stress.[1] You go see the doctor, you explain your situation, and what does the doctor do? *Chances are, he or she writes out a prescription.*

But that prescription usually only masks the *symptoms* of stress. It's not addressing what may be causing those symptoms in the first place. As a naïve player in this scenario, you may believe the prescription has wiped out the problem, because you no longer have any symptoms. This can happen when treating such (potentially) stress-related health problems as migraine headaches, anxiety, allergies, recurrent colds and gastro-intestinal problems.

And this happens quite frequently when treating insomnia because approximately 50% of all insomnia *is caused by stress.*[2] So, if you go to your doctor and tell him or her you're not sleeping well, chances are you will go back home with a prescription for an insomnia medication. But that pill isn't going to take away the toxic boss or the difficult relationship or the financial stress you are dealing with because you've just been laid off from your job or a pandemic has arrived or your elderly mother is in need of constant care and you are the only one who can provide it. So, if stress is what's keeping you up at night, the pill is simply masking a symptom (i.e., sleeplessness) of stress.

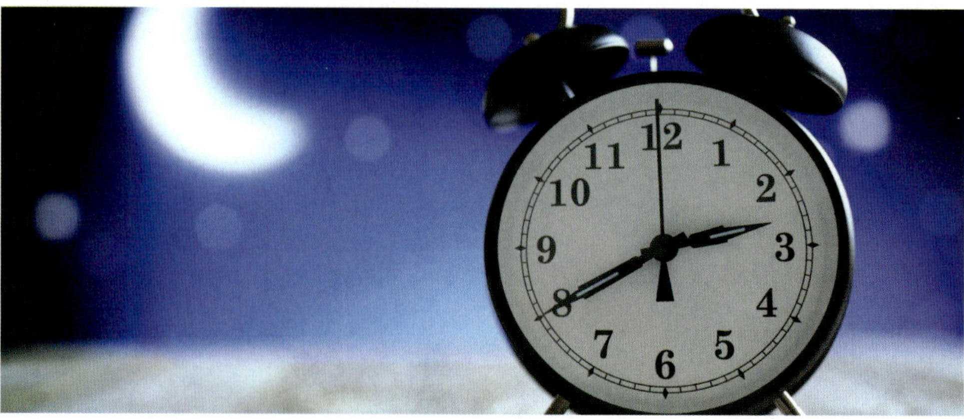

What's worse, your prescription is allowing you to ignore your stress while it silently builds over weeks and months and sometimes even years. If this unrelenting stress goes on for long enough, it can result in medical problems that are much worse than the initial symptoms that drove you to the doctor in the first place. These symptoms might have been easily dealt with from the get-go, if you had addressed the causes of your stress RATHER THAN JUST THE SYMPTOMS! Depression, anxiety, high blood pressure and heart disease are just a few of the health problems that chronic stress can lead to.

There's another reason to consider stress reduction (which includes mindfulness meditation) as your best defense against stress-related DIS-EASE: *It has no side effects.* **Take a look at the common side effects of a popular insomnia medication called Halcion.[3] (Taken from RX.com) These side effects include:**

- Dizziness
- Tiredness
- Loss of coordination
- Headaches
- Depression
- Memory problems
- Numbness
- Nervousness
- Excitability
- Irritability
- Changes in menstrual cycles
- Itching
- Decreased interest in sex
- Blurred vision

Now look at what this same site regards as the "serious side effects" of Halcion:

Tell your doctor if you have serious side effects of Halcion including memory loss, or mental/mood/behavior changes (such as new or worsening depression, abnormal thoughts, thoughts of suicide, hallucinations, confusion, agitation, aggressive behavior, or anxiety).

And now look at what this same site regards as the uncommon side-effects.

Rarely, after taking Halcion, people have gotten out of bed and driven vehicles while not fully awake ("sleep-driving"). People have also sleepwalked, prepared/eaten food, made phone calls, or had sex while not fully awake. Often, these people do not remember these events. This problem can be dangerous to you or to others. If you find out that you have done any of these activities after taking Halcion, tell your doctor right away.

Are you prepared to put up with even the CHANCE of any of these side effects for what amounts to about 20-30 minutes of EXTRA SLEEP on average for those taking all forms of insomnia medication?[4]

Full disclosure: mindfulness meditation does have one major side effect: It may cause you to fall asleep.

When doctors graduate from medical school they take a 2000-year old oath that goes all the way back to a physician named Hippocrates who was practicing medicine in ancient Greece. That sacred vow says simply: "First, do no harm." Known as the Hippocratic Oath, this oath is really a promise NOT to engage in any form of quackery. In other words, doctors must NOT run the risk of prescribing medicines or suggesting procedures that do more harm than good. Fortunately, most pharmaceutical solutions have been tested thoroughly and are proven to do more GOOD than harm. None-the-less, all drugs have certain side effects.

Many of the patients who first came to The Mindfulness-based stress reduction clinic, were dealing with chronic pain. And of course, most were being treated – unsuccessfully – with pain medications. Pain medications often work for a while, and then require stronger and stronger doses to work successfully. But these gradually increasing dosages lead to dependency and addiction. Fast forward 40 years to today, and it's easy to see, the problems that were created by relying way too heavily on prescriptive approaches to pain has only exacerbated the problem.

I grew up in Connecticut not far from the Town of Lyme. Lyme, Connecticut, in case you didn't know, is ground zero for Lyme disease. That's where it first appeared in the US and that's how it got its name. Living in Connecticut, all my life, I apparently had Lyme early on, before anyone knew what it was.

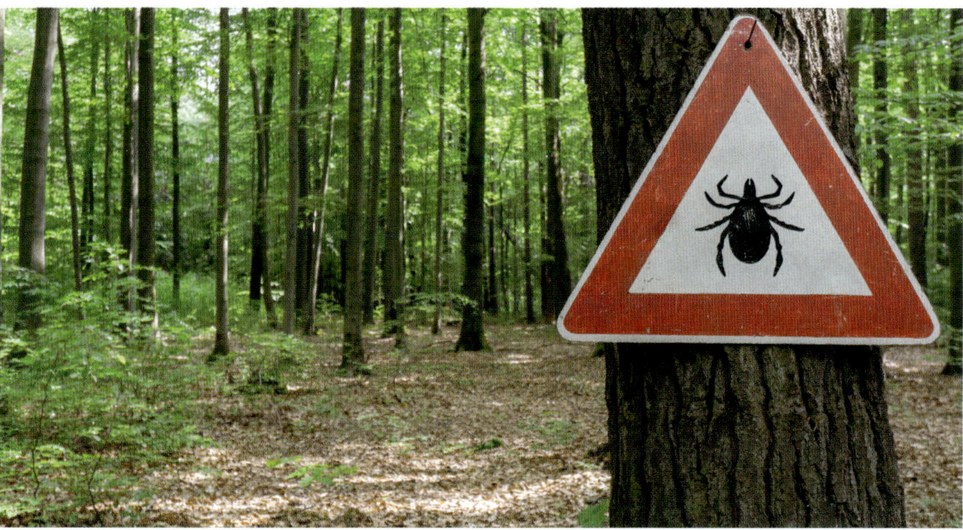

I remember in my twenties, getting this recurring pain in my thighs. But it only really bothered me during the changeover (in temperature) from fall to winter and then again, from winter to spring. I just coped with the pain as best I could. I'd take a couple of ibuprofens a day during the most difficult days and tough it out on other days. Of course, *the ibuprofen wasn't addressing the root of the problem*, it was just taking away the symptoms of my Lyme disease.

When I turned 40 the pain started to occur year-round. By this time, everyone in Connecticut knew what Lyme was, so I finally went to the doctor and got tested. While I was waiting for the results to come back from the lab, the pain got so intense, I was taking 10-20 ibuprofen a day. (A major side effect of ibuprofen is heartburn, so I was taking Prilosec as well to manage my symptoms of heart burn. Another common problem with prescriptive – and over the counter solutions is: *Taking pills to treat the side effects of the pills you are already taking.*)

My doctor, an infectious disease specialist, asked me on my return visit if I liked gardening and/or hiking in the woods. When I answered yes to both, she said something that really surprised me. "You are just like my husband. I get him tested every year. He's had Lyme 13 times."

Aren't you glad you don't live in Connecticut?

She suggested a heavy one-month long treatment with a very strong antibiotic to knock out the Lyme. I remember being completely pain-free for the first time in years. In this case, the pharmaceutical approach worked perfectly. Why? Because the medicine I was taking was knocking out a specific infectious disease. It WAS addressing the root of the problem.

At Jon Kabat-Zinn's clinic many of the clients were coming in for help with pain management. As is so often the case, the source of a patient's pain isn't as easy to pinpoint as it was for my case with Lyme disease. And that's why The Center for Mindfulness was able to help patients no one else could. Pain is often the result of inflammation. Stress causes inflammation. Meditation, yoga, exercise and eating lots of fruits and veggies helps control it.

If you have issues around pain, particularly now - in light of all the problems with addiction to pain medications – your doctor will probably encourage you to consider *alternative* approaches, rather than quickly prescribing a narcotic pain medication. Try meditating and see what happens, he or she might say. "It won't do you any harm."

This is a key piece of information you need to know about the various forms of stress management we are talking about in this book, whether it's mindfulness meditation, progressive muscle relaxation, biofeedback or deep breathing. They could very well relieve the problem, but they certainly won't make it worse. Especially if you approach these alternative solutions with your doctor's permission and guidance: Because these approaches come with ZERO side effects.

Holistic, or alternative, or as health care systems like to call it, *integrative* medicine, CAN promise to first do no harm, especially if you use these approaches in tandem with whatever approaches your doctor might be recommending. That's why the preferred term now is integrative medicine. You *integrate* the holistic solution along *with* other mainstream approaches your doctor might recommend.

In a mindfulness study done on two groups of patients with psoriasis, one group got the standard light therapy. The other group got the standard light therapy PLUS an eight-week Mindfulness course. The mindfulness group recovered from their psoriasis twice as fast as those who got the usual treatment alone. This is a great example of how integrative medicine can work in tandem with mainstream medicine.[5]

But when it comes to problems with anxiety, depression and even gastro-intestinal issues like IBS, you might want to do a little research on your own, before seeing your doctor. For example, with depression, Cognitive Behavioral Therapy has been shown to be as effective as medication in treating depression and in some cases, more effective.[6] Even the Journal of the American Medical Association (JAMA) reported that anti-depressants "*are no better than a placebo at treating mild to moderate cases of depression.*"[7]

And yet, most doctors will quickly prescribe an anti-depressant – despite a long list of side effects, perhaps even more impressive than the side effects listed above for Halcion – because they've seen it alleviate depression rather quickly in so many cases. Here is where YOU must be very knowledgeable in order to obtain the treatment that works best for you.

Most people are surprised to learn that, for treating many mental health issues, a placebo (AKA a sugar pill) is sometimes (as reported in JAMA) as effective as a real pill. For

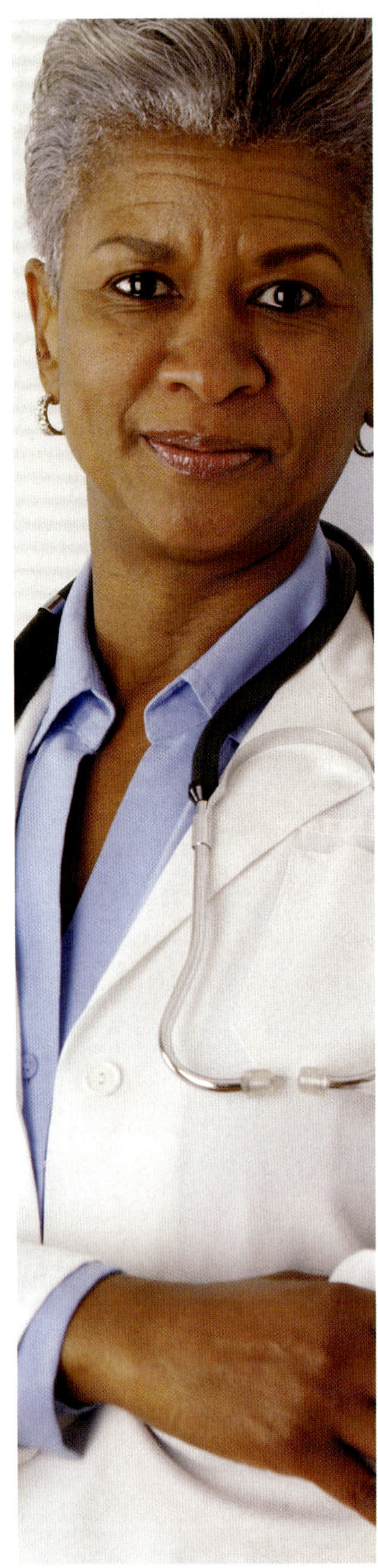

a prescription medicine to be approved by the FDA, it only needs to be slightly *more* effective than a placebo. Why? Because doctors can't ethically prescribe a placebo even though they've been show to work about 40 to 50% of the time. Your doctor's only option is to prescribe a real pill and that often comes with side effects.

So, while you are taking your prescription, also engaging in practices like mindfulness meditation, yoga, exercise, and healthy eating is going to significantly improve the odds of your recovery. If your problem goes away, *and your doctor agrees*, you may get to the point where you can reduce the dosage or try going off of the medication entirely. For people with health problems like rashes and asthma and autoimmune disorders that are sometimes made worse by the medications, finding a doctor who will help you consider alternative approaches – in addition to your pharmaceutical options - can save you months and months, sometimes even years, of going down the wrong road, in order to find a solution to your stress-related health problem.

One of the most famous doctors of the last century, Albert Schweitzer, once said, "*Each patient carries their own doctor inside of him. We are at our best when we allow this doctor to do its work.*"[10] In other words, the body ultimately heals itself and doctors can only hope to facilitate that process.

So, you want to find a doctor who is committed to helping YOU facilitate your own healing process. With that said, remember, during the average office visit, your primary care physician has about 7-8 minutes to diagnose your condition. He or she, may not have the time to get into the intricacies (or subtleties) of your condition, *especially if it involves stress.*

For example, if you were to go to the doctor with a skin rash in the spring or summer, he or she is probably going to ask: have you been out in the woods, or out gardening? If your answer is yes, he or she might assume that you have come in contact with poison ivy. In which case, you might be prescribed a cortisone cream. If you really did touch poison ivy, that cortisone cream will often work like a charm.

But if your rash is caused in part by stress, and NOT by touching poison ivy, guess what? You will be applying a man-made stress chemical to the surface of your skin that just might make the problem worse.

There used to be an advertisement for a discount clothing store in the greater New York area. Their tag line was: *An educated consumer is our best customer.* This chapter is meant to encourage you to become an educated consumer when it comes to your health. Learn as much as you can about your condition, BEFORE going to see the doctor. Learn about stress and stress related disease. Learn about side effects from common medications that you are taking or that might be prescribed. And, most importantly, ask your doctor point blank if the medications that you will be taking are in fact, treating the source of the problem or just taking away the symptoms.

You are ALREADY educating yourself about alternative solutions to stress related health problems and know, that when you pursue these solutions in an integrated way with whatever your doctor is prescribing, these approaches won't do you any harm and they might do you a whole lot of good.

That's why, from its humble beginnings in Shrewsbury, Massachusetts, The Center for Mindfulness now has programs offered in hundreds of hospitals throughout the US and Canada. And these clinics are showing patients new non-invasive, non-prescriptive, non-addicting solutions for dealing with chronic pain, depression, anxiety, immune system problems, eating disorders, PTSD, alcoholism, drug addiction and more.[11] All with absolutely no side effects, except one: *You might fall asleep while meditating.**

*Since writing this chapter, I have seen some research, published in Dan Goleman and Richard Davidson's book ALTERED TRAITS, that for people who have suffered from trauma, mindfulness meditation, in certain cases can be troubling, because it can bring back memories that person might not be ready to face.

The Amazing Power of Placebos

The placebo effect is an amazingly complex phenomenon with lots of subtle nuances. In certain studies, researchers have learned they can no longer give out plain sugar pills that have no side-effects because if there are no side effects, the people in the "control group" know they are getting the placebo, and this can compromise the results of the study. So, they create pills with harmless side effects.

In other studies where these sugar pills are still being used, the participants taking the placebo often complain bitterly of side effects they are suffering from when there are no side effects.

Recently, researchers wanted to see if a certain kind of knee surgery for a meniscus tear was truly effective, so a study was conducted involving placebo surgery. All the participants in the study had a torn meniscus. Half the patients got the real surgery and the other half got the placebo surgery which involved making tiny incisions that matched the arthroscopic incisions of the real surgery. The group with the placebo surgery fared as well or better than the group with the real surgery.[8]

Placebos really speak to the power of belief and the power of the mind to heal the body. There is now some research that indicates, even when your doctor tells you: "I'm giving you a placebo" that it can still be effective, as long as the doctor explains that placebos really work and this might actually make you feel better.[9] This level of transparency would open the doors for doctors actually PRESCRIBING a placebo.

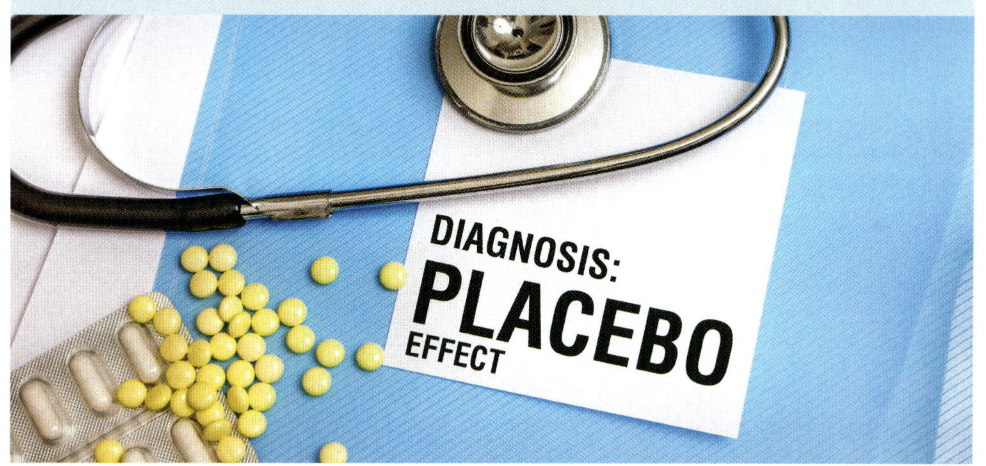

Chapter 8

Mindfulness and Depression

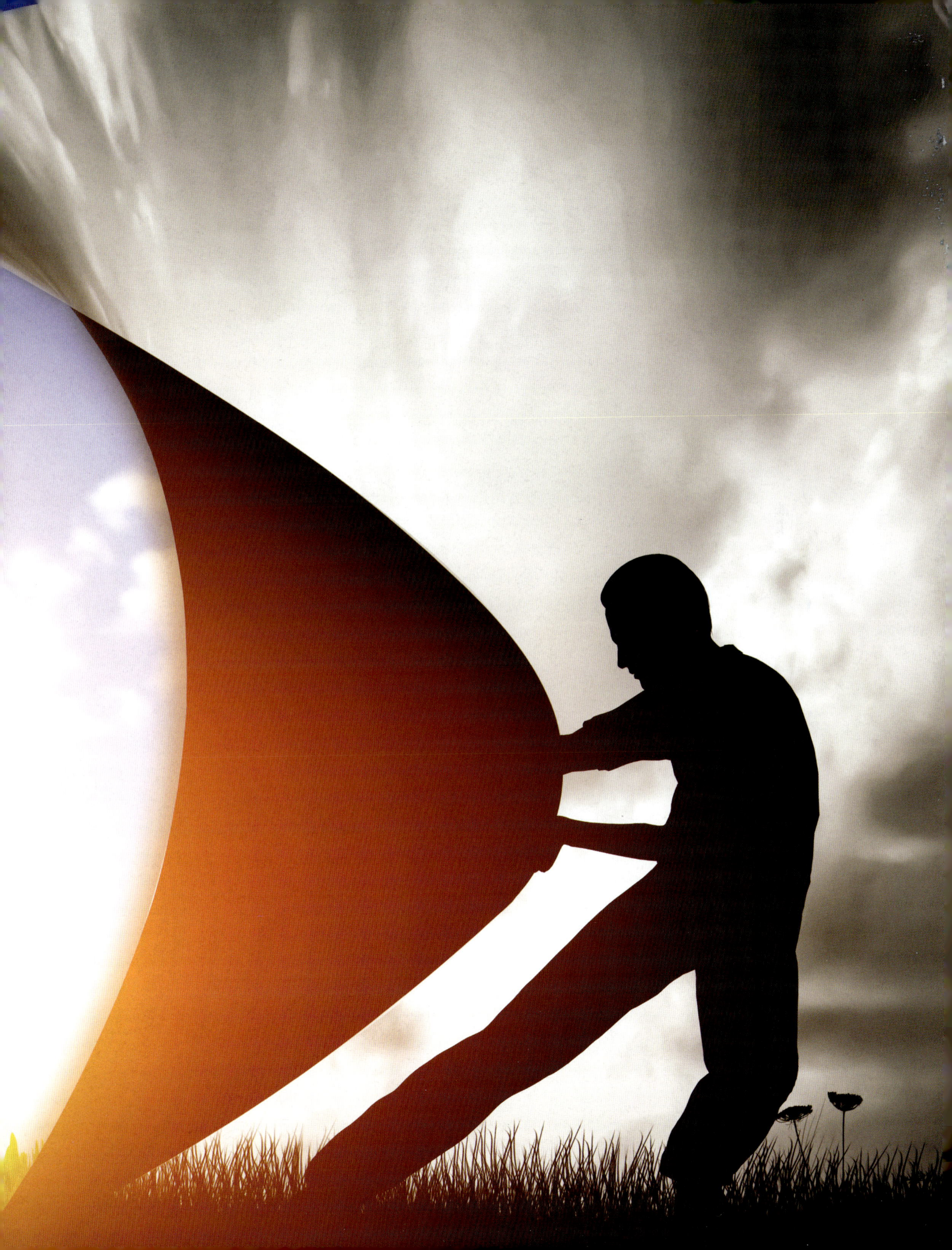

Chapter 8
Mindfulness and Depression

Getting well is only half the problem, staying well is the other half.

For those who have battled depression - now, along with stress, considered an epidemic by the World Health Organization - the biggest issue for many people is *relapse.* Each bout of clinical depression dramatically increases the likelihood of yet another bout.[1] One bout gives way to another, and soon any hope of lifting one's self out of depression becomes less and less likely.

"People with clinical depression become increasingly difficult to treat with each successive bout they experience," explains Dr. Bruce McEwen, stress expert and professor at Rockefeller University, "Up to 50% of depression cases are now considered treatment resistant."[2]

Any person who has ever suffered from depression, and this includes me, knows that even after you get better, any time you experience even a short episode of sadness, you WORRY whether this temporary state of sadness is going to drag you down into another *prolonged* state of sadness, i.e., depression. A lot of people start taking antidepressants, get over their depression, but never stop taking the pills because they are so afraid of falling back into depression again.

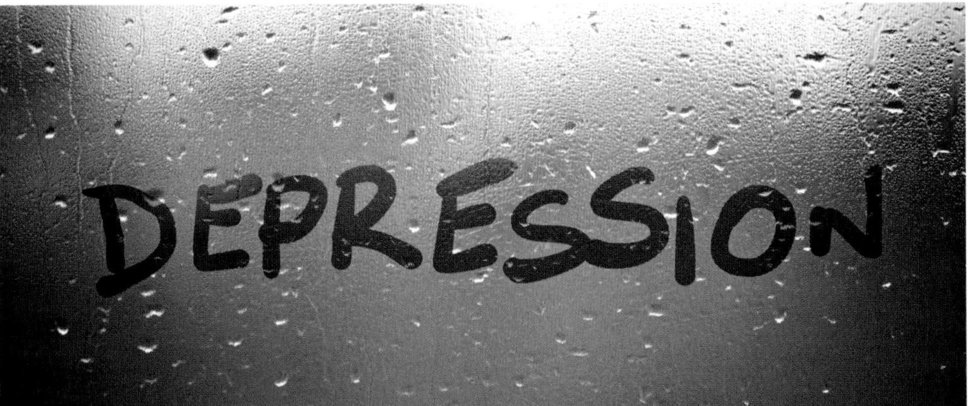

Canadian scientist, Dr. Zindel Segal's mindful approach to treating depression, called Mindfulness Based Cognitive Restructuring (MBCT) not only helps patients who have relapsed more than once, it helps them maintain their recovery, too. And sometimes, without need of medication.

When Segal first started looking at depression in the early 1990's there had been dramatic progress in treating it. At the time, newly introduced anti-depressants seemed to be helping people recover from depression, and studies of cognitive behavioral therapy, looked promising too. Despite all this progress in treating the disease, relapse was still a major issue. As Segal often says: "*Getting well is only half the problem. Staying well is the other half.*"[3]

In his search for an answer to how to prevent relapse, Segal learned about a study that followed patients who continued taking their medication for two years after fully recovering. The study showed that this simple difference (of continuing to take their meds) had prevented relapse in those patients. But there was still one big problem with this seemingly simple solution to the problem of relapse. Many patients stop taking their depression medications as soon as they feel better due to side effects like weight gain, lack of sex drive, cost and other issues.

Segal had tried transcendental meditation in college, as had several of the others on his team, but none of them had a regular practice of meditating or had even considered it as a way of helping patients with depression. That's about the time they ran into the work of Dr. Marsha Linehan.

Linehan is the founder of a form of therapy called Dialectical Behavioral Therapy or DBT (which includes aspects of mindfulness). Back then, Linehan was trying to help her clients deal with addiction problems and borderline personality disorder which most therapists at the time thought couldn't be helped with *any* form of treatment.

Until Dr. Linehan came along, no one had come up with a solution to the delicate problem of how to tell an addict that their behavior was bad, but as individuals they were OK. In other words, patients would equate hearing about their bad behavior (drug-taking and cutting) with being a bad person. Even though this wasn't the intent of the therapist, it still came across that way to the patient. When that would happen, patients didn't last very long in therapy: Feeling bad about themselves, they would typically slip back into their familiar pattern of taking drugs to soothe themselves for feeling bad.

Linehan realized that she had to come up with a way of supporting behavior change while propping up the patient at the same time. (The word *dialectical* refers to addressing these two opposing forces.) Her form of counseling had to assist the patient in realizing that they could still be a good person even if their outward behavior was considered bad. By teaching patients the mindfulness ideas of accepting where they were in recovery *unconditionally,* and being able to see their *behavior* as separate from who they were as people, this allowed formerly untreatable patients to embrace the therapeutic intervention Linehan was offering, rather than reject it.

Naturally her work with these clients – which was having an unheard-of success rate - attracted the attention of many people in the field including Dr. Segal.[4] He was traveling regularly down to Boston from Canada to meet with her to learn more. Both he and Linehan were interested in helping patients avoid the self-harm that often goes with undiagnosed cases of depression, and in Linehan's case, borderline personality disorder. Linehan suggested that Segal and his fellow researchers get in touch with, at that point, a little-known author and mindfulness expert named Jon Kabat-Zinn.

Segal and his group got a copy of Kabat-Zinn's first book: "Full Catastrophe Living" and started reading it. Immediately, they began to see some ways that this approach to helping people recover from all kinds of health problems, including chronic pain, might also help patients avoid relapsing into depression.

The key feature was how mindfulness could help people detach from their thoughts and their emotions. Segal illustrates this point beautifully in his lectures with a diagram of a spiral – think spiraling down into depression - that links thoughts like "*I'm a bad parent*" and "*I'm not good at anything*" on one side of the spiral to corresponding emotions like *sadness, guilt and shame on the other*. Each thought, *when tied to the corresponding emotion*, has the potential to drag a person down the spiral further and further into sadness and depression.[5]

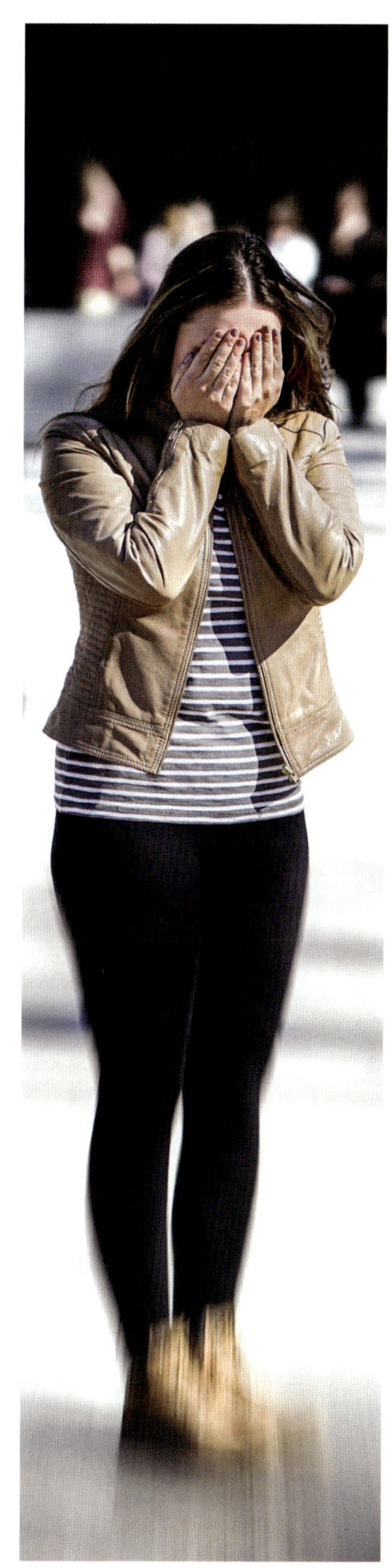

What helped me get out of depression.

Three things really helped move me forward in my journey to long-lasting recovery from depression:

1. People who revealed their own struggles with depression. This included actor Jim Carrey, former football star Terry Bradshaw and even the behavioral change specialist Dr. James Prochaska. A couple of close friends of mine revealed it too. There was so much stigma around this issue back then that all these people, my friends included, were quite brave – even daring - to go public with their personal struggles with depression. Suddenly, I didn't feel so alone.

2. A book entitled "Lincoln's Melancholy" by Joshua Wolf Shenk. Shenk wrote about how the world took a different view toward melancholy (i.e., depression) in Abraham Lincoln's day. This characteristic was to be expected in a person if you wanted someone who was a deep thinker. People like Lincoln and Winston Churchill, who also suffered from depression, were deep thinkers and people that I greatly admired.

3. Mindfulness. The idea that you could distance yourself from overly negative thoughts and emotions. As I got better and better at this, I got more and more confident about my ability to prevent myself from relapsing into depression. Eventually I stopped worrying whether occasional bouts of sadness would drag me back into another prolonged episode of what Winston Churchill nicknamed "the black dog."

What initially looked so appealing to Segal and his group was that mindfulness could help people detach thoughts from emotions and free them from this downward spiral. Their studies had specifically shown that the ability of a patient to deal with sadness after recovery from depression (and be able to detach from it) had a great deal to do with whether they would relapse or whether they wouldn't. Training in mindfulness might provide the key to avoiding relapse.

In my own personal battle with depression, I remember reading Dr. David Burns' book The New Mood Therapy and seeing how cognitive therapy had helped a lot of people recover from depression. While a lot of the tools and tricks of cognitive therapy had helped me enormously, they still didn't completely free me from this battle.

Albert Ellis, one of the cofounders of Cognitive Behavioral Therapy or CBT, liked to say that once you become aware that you are having an irrational thought, all you have to do is change it.[6] I ran into one simple problem with this instruction that turned out to be quite profound. There were times when I knew my thinking was irrational, *but there was nothing I could do to change it.* For example, when you feel like a failure, even though your life has been full of success, you suddenly realize that the mind is capable of taking you down at any moment no matter how aware you are that your thinking is irrational. Zindel Segal's work gave me the confidence to KNOW that I could overcome this weakness in CBT.

Generally, as human beings we turn away from sadness and suffering. We try to sweep it under the rug, particularly symptoms like anxiety and depression. Nobody needs to know about this, we say to ourselves, and we try to pretend like nothing is wrong. Mindfulness takes a different tack. It suggests that you go toward the suffering and the pain and mentally *confront* it by becoming mindful of it.

It's the thinking mind that generates the thoughts that in turn, generate these sad feelings. With mindful awareness, you can train yourself to just watch – with a certain amount of detachment – these negative thoughts and the emotions created by the thoughts. When you watch them carefully from a distance, you will see how they often seem to diminish and suddenly disappear almost like a soap bubble that pops, right in front of your eyes, for no apparent reason.

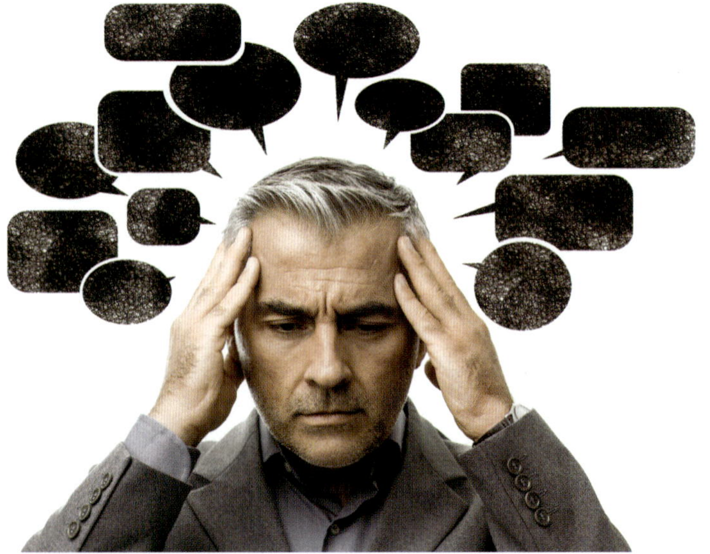

There was one more step in helping figure out how to prevent relapse in people who had suffered bouts of clinical depression. Zindel Segal and his colleagues, Drs. Mark Williams and John Teasdale, needed to devise an intervention that could induce *a temporary state of sadness.* This intervention would help them discover those people most likely to relapse.

The team had their potential subjects watch one of the closing scenes from the movie "Terms of Endearment." If you've never seen this movie, (it won the Academy award for Best Picture) it's all about a 40-something woman, played by Debra Winger, who is dying of cancer. (Up until this point, the movie is a comedy which costars Jack Nicholson and Shirley MacLaine.) In this final scene, where the movie turns suddenly tragic, Winger's character tries to give her young son a pep-talk about going on without her. The actor who plays this part, is *really* crying, and Debra Winger is crying, and you, the viewer, inevitably wind up crying too.

In their research, Segal and his colleagues found that the people most affected by this scene were ALSO *the most likely to relapse back into depression.* (I ALWAYS cry when I see this scene.) Knowing this, the authors had to come up with a specific technique that could help depression sufferers deal with similar moments of sadness which – as their research had shown – were like incubators for relapse back into depression. (CBT was great for getting people out of depression, but it was not as helpful at preventing relapse BACK into depression.)

As Segal points out again and again: with depression, recovery is only half the battle. Depression is episodic so a patient also needs a set of tools to help him or her get through their future moments of sadness once the initial treatment is over. "Sadness is a symptom of depression, but when people are no longer depressed, sadness can bring to mind judgmental, critical and harsh ways of thinking about, and viewing oneself, that can sometimes tip people over the edge into a new episode of depression."[7] Thus, if there was something that could help these patients navigate the sad moments in life like these, then relapse prevention might be achieved.

"But how do you work with a trigger like sadness when sadness is a key feature of our universal human experience?" Segal asked at a lecture I attended at the Center for Mindfulness in Shrewsbury, Massachusetts. "We weren't interested in trying to eliminate sadness or trying to get people not to feel sad. What we were really interested in doing was helping people develop a different relationship to their sadness. And that's why mindfulness turned out to be the perfect solution."[8]

CBT says that all emotions are predicated by thoughts. But we now know that this isn't always true. Sometimes emotions generate thoughts. And when this happens it's much harder to simply change an irrational thought. Mindfulness says you don't have to change it, *you simply change your relationship to it.*

One of the guiding principles of mindfulness is: you are not your thoughts.

There's a great bumper sticker that says just about the same thing: *You don't have to believe everything you think.* When you have self-destructive thoughts, brought on by a period of sadness, instead of giving way to it, you can step back, and realize that this is the thinking mind, doing what the thinking mind often does: Spinning out yarns that may have a grain of truth but are mostly just pure fiction.

Most people who become depressed have nervous systems that have become dysregulated. When the brain becomes dysregulated, the amygdala grows bigger and becomes MORE sensitive to stress. The more sensitive to stress we become the more likely we are to get depressed. When we practice self-regulation techniques like mindfulness meditation, areas of the pre-frontal cortex get bigger while the amygdala grows smaller.[9] This ability to self-regulate the nervous system is the secret sauce, if you will, when it comes to using mindfulness to combat depression. The patient is using mindfulness in a way that not only wins the battle for recovery but also helps win the war of avoiding relapse.

The battle can be short-lived, but the war is lifelong. And mindfulness is a strategy that has been proven to work long term. Here you are using a simple mind-body technique, like staying in the present moment while detaching yourself from your overly negative thinking to create permanent, structural changes in the brain that can give you the power to avoid falling into a second or third bout of what eventually becomes untreatable depression.

People who suffer from depression often have trouble with rumination, where they spend an inordinate amount of time trapped in their thinking mind. But by tapping into sensation, or what Segal calls "the present moment awareness pathway," people are freed from the thinking mind trap. Segal instructs patients to notice their senses: What does the chair feel like? What does the flower smell like? What does a cricket sound like? This pathway through sensations reverts back to the insula – a part of the brain responsible for empathy and self-compassion – which allows us to pause our thoughts long enough to regain control of them – especially at crucial times when these thoughts are spiraling *out of control.*

Add in the detached awareness, which allows us to just observe what's happening, along with this focus on sensation, and suddenly we are able to cope with sadness without letting it overwhelm us. Sadness becomes a *temporary* feeling that in most cases, will go away, if we let it. Tapping into the present moment pathway can help us do that.

One last thought about mindfulness and depression. People who practice mindfulness feel a sense of reward for engaging in that practice. One of the hallmarks of depression is a condition psychologists call *anhedonia*, where the things that once brought you pleasure, and you found rewarding, no longer do. Mindfulness helps bring back this love of pleasure and reward and thus *makes a person want to keep doing it*. In this important way, mindfulness practice becomes self-perpetuating. And that may be the most important reason why mindfulness helps people avoid relapse back into depression.

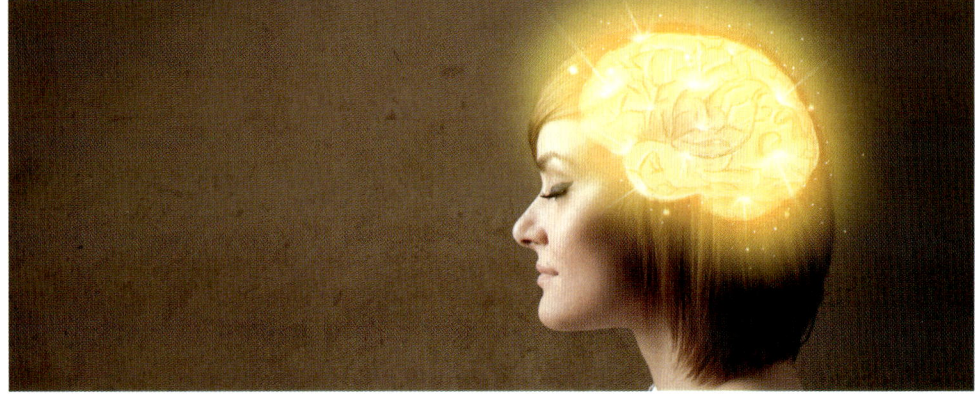

Opening the present moment pathway.

When you THINK ABOUT the world, your information comes to you by an indirect pathway. This indirect way of retrieving information about the world comes loaded with biases, interpretations, judgments, expectations and beliefs, all of which can sometimes make you feel depressed and sad.

You can't even see a blade of crab grass without judging it through this interpretive pathway. (Crab grass is bad.) But by opening ourselves up to direct perception of the world through our senses, we experience the world with less judgment, with less emotion and with fewer preconceived notions about how the world ought or ought not to be.

Every time you touch something really soft, smell something really fragrant, or taste something really wonderful, or see something really magnificent, your present moment pathway opens up and FREES you momentarily from the tyranny of the thinking mind. This brief moment of freedom is sometimes just enough to get you over certain sad moments that come up in everyday life. It's just that depressed people have more difficulty navigating these moments. The present moment pathway gives you a guidance system to help steer your ship through the rough waters of occasional sadness.

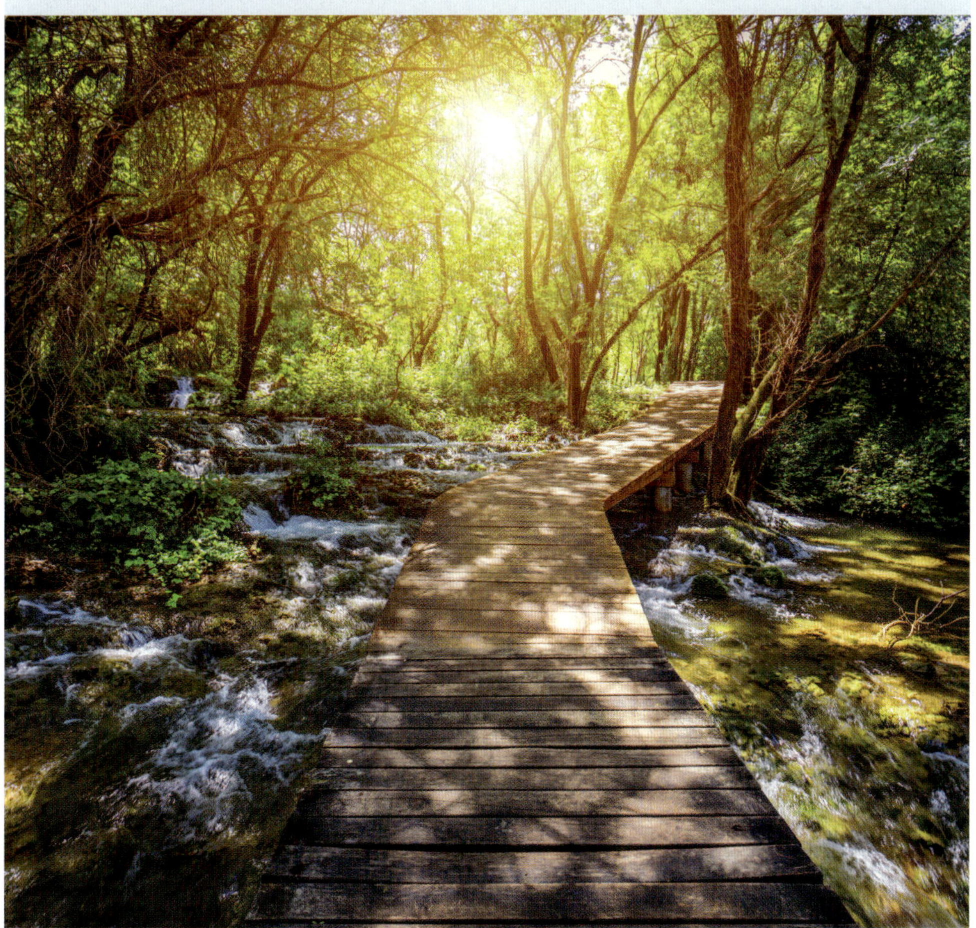

Chapter 9

Mindfulness and Addiction

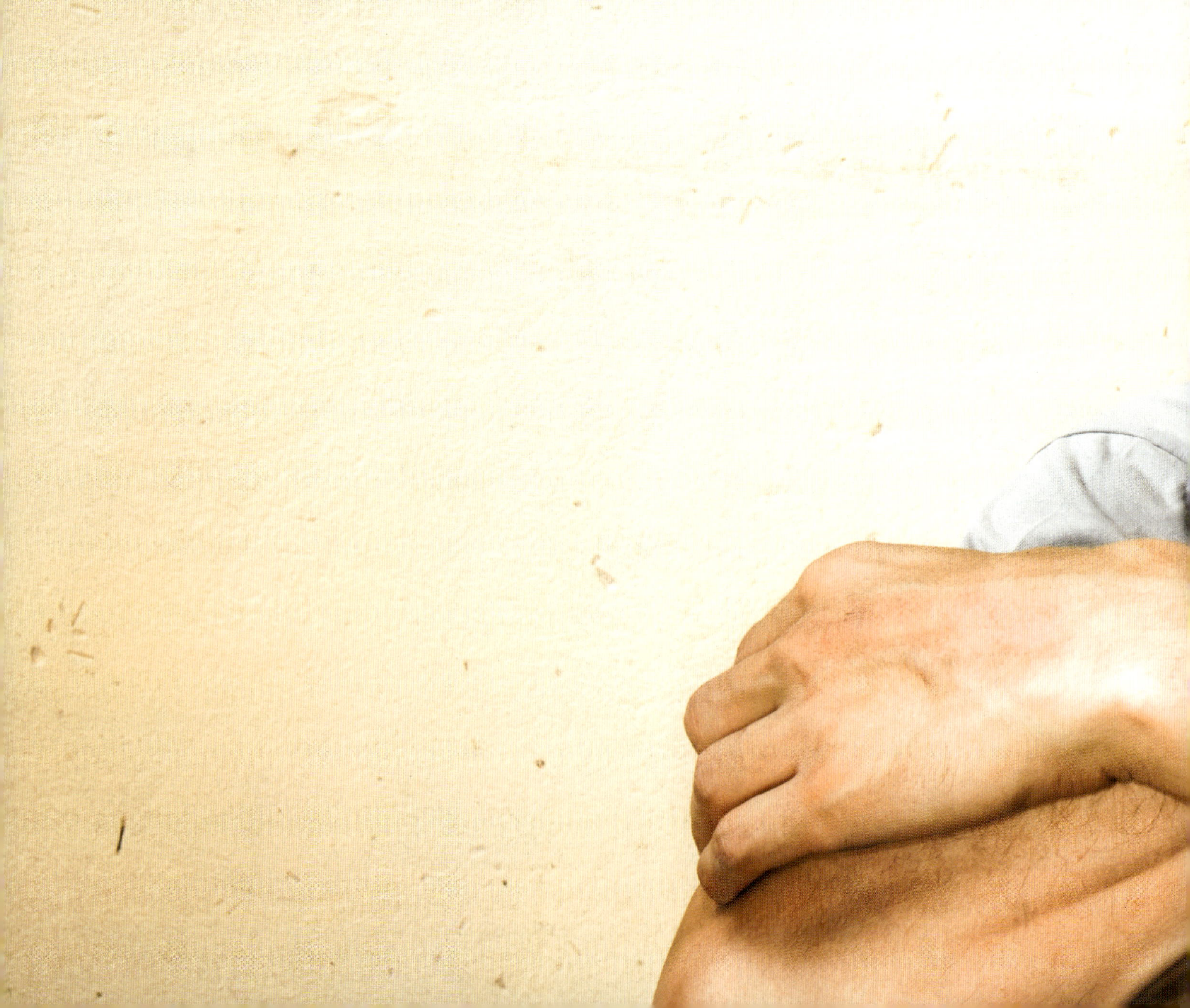

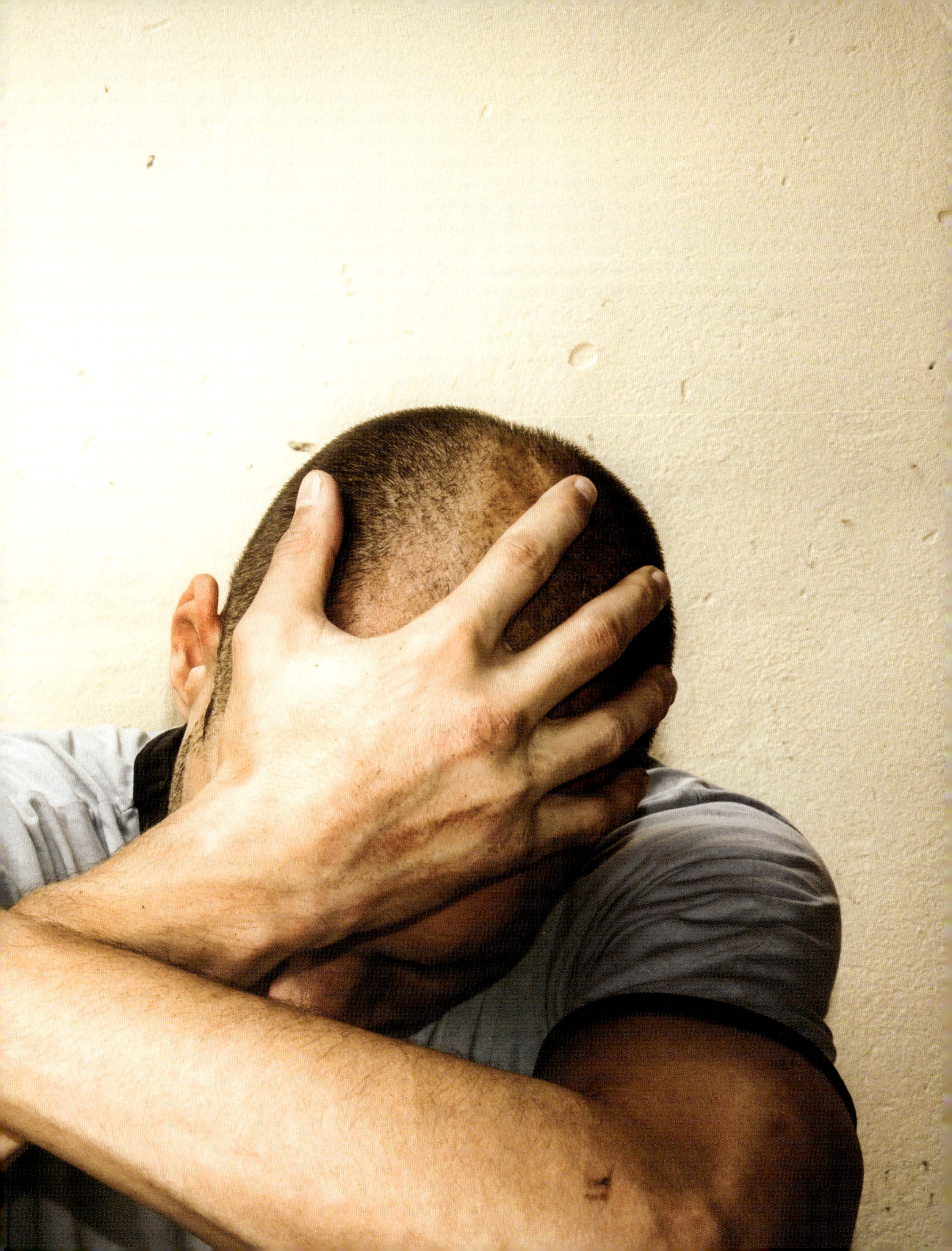

Dr. James Prochaska's Stages of Change (for smoking cessation)

Precontemplation
Thinking about giving up smoking but not quite ready yet.

Contemplation
Learning about why one should quit and how.

Preparation
Choosing a plan of action (patch, smoking cessation class, etc.)

Action
Putting the plan into action.

Maintenance
Relapsing 4-5 times before finally quitting.

Termination
No longer tempted by the old habit.

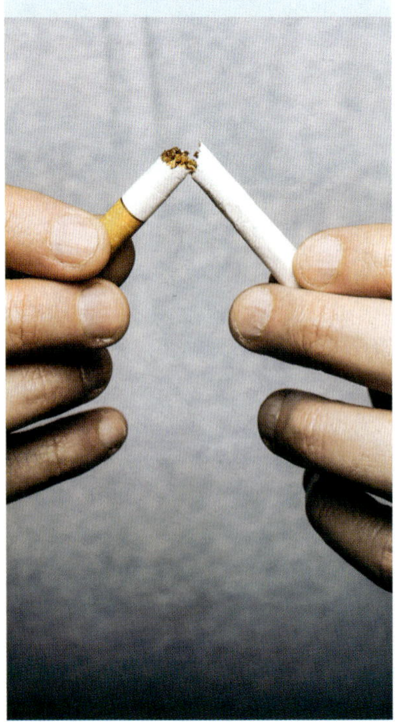

Chapter 9
Mindfulness and Addiction

Judson Brewer, M.D, has developed an interesting approach to teaching people how to quit smoking. "Go ahead and smoke all you want," Dr. Brewer tells his clients. "Just do it mindfully." Brewer, director of The Mindfulness Center at Brown University, is teaching people how to tackle all sorts of addictions with mindfulness, not just smoking. Brewer talks about how people have addictions to Facebook, Instagram, smart phones, TV, food, not to mention drugs and alcohol which are the terms more commonly associated with the idea of addiction. But Brewer defines addiction simply as "continuous use despite adverse consequences."[1]

When smokers come into his program, and begin to smoke mindfully, they start to see their habit differently. He quotes one woman who said, "When I smoke now it smells like chemicals and tastes like stinky cheese."

As Brewer puts it: *We HACK the cycle of craving and reward that leads to ALL addictions.* That cycle goes like this: We feel BAD (for whatever reason), we CRAVE something that will make the bad feeling go away (like a cigarette or a piece of chocolate cake) and when we allow ourselves to HAVE what we want, we feel better. In a nutshell, that's the cycle of craving and addiction![2]

That's a very hard cycle to break.

But when a smoker begins to see – in a very real, visceral way that smoking is NOT a reward, that new way of thinking, begins to break the cycle. In other words, instead of trying to change a smoker's thoughts and beliefs about their addiction (which would be a cognitive-behavioral approach), Brewer is using the *smoker's own observations* about what smoking really feels like, to get them to internally WANT to quit.[3]

That's how you HACK the cycle.

He shares other anecdotes about clients who, after they start to smoke mindfully, realize that smoking tastes really bad: "It tastes like dirt." "It tastes terrible," they report. Mindfulness expert Dr. John Weaver says the same thing about eating a McDonald's hamburger: "Don't try eating a piece of a McDonald's hamburger mindfully. You'll regret it!"

Behavioral change expert Dr. James Prochaska's research on smoking cessation helps us understand why old-fashioned approaches to overcoming addiction don't work. People quit gradually, in stages. Outdated models expected smokers to quit cold turkey. Giving up their cigarettes overnight - without considering the stages they usually go through on their way to giving it up entirely. Brewer's advice to smoke mindfully is another way to address this same issue.

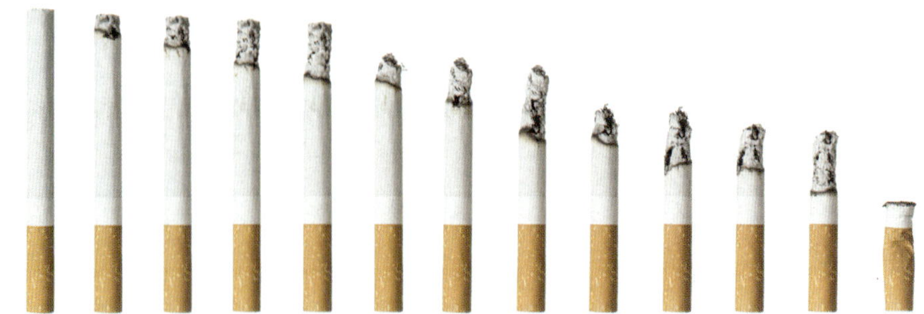

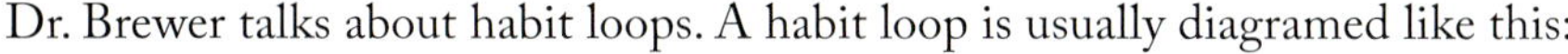

Dr. Brewer talks about habit loops. A habit loop is usually diagramed like this:

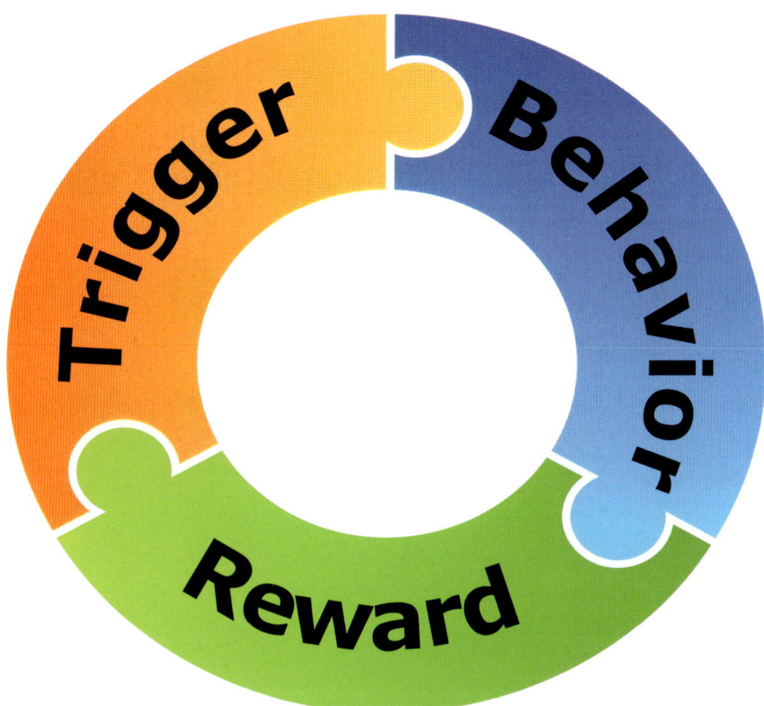

In the above diagram – especially when we are talking about addiction - the reward starts the whole cycle over again. This is what leads to addiction.

Here's a habit loop we ALL can relate to:

You feel stressed > You eat a cookie > You feel better.

But now that you know eating a cookie makes you feel better (at least in the short term), you want another cookie! And you may want a cookie in lots of different situations because your trigger here is any source of stress. This is what you learn in Introduction to Psychology Class. It's called operant conditioning. Harvard psychologist BF Skinner applied this model to small animals in cages. A light in the cage flashes (Trigger), the rat or pigeon presses a bar (Behavior), and it gets a food pellet (Reward). Rats and pigeons will press the bar thousands of times if the trigger is powerful enough. (A drop of dopamine, for example can cause this kind of overwhelming response.)[4]

Here's where habit loops get interesting and a bit confusing. Whether the initial cue or trigger is positive (you get a promotion) or negative (you get fired) in either case, *you still crave the cookie*! Once you've learned a habit loop where doing a certain thing – like eating a cookie, or a piece of chocolate cake, or smoking a cigarette - makes you feel better, you may do it whether your trigger or cue is pleasant or unpleasant. The cue may be seeing a fresh-baked cookie in a store (pleasant) or it may be getting chewed out by your boss (unpleasant); Either event may leave you craving a cookie.[5]

Sustainable Behavioral Change

Michelle Segar, Ph.D., is a behavioral change scientist at the University of Michigan. She says changing your behavior is all about finding the right whys. In order to get motivated: "Health is not the right hook. Thirty minutes of moving is not about thirty minutes of moving," she explains. "It's about the other 23 ½ hours a day. It's when we move more, and have more energy, and reduce our stress that we enjoy work more, we're more patient parents, we don't snap at our spouses (quite so much), and it enhances our whole day. That's the hook."[8]

Michelle Segar's approach is a mindfulness approach: Because it's all about how you feel right now, not years from now.

So, when you think about making behavior changes like giving up smoking, changing your diet, exercising more, or starting a meditation practice, spend some time thinking about what the right whys might be for you. Whether that's having more energy, feeling better, sleeping better, focusing more easily or being able to spend more quality time with friends and family, these are just some examples of the kinds of immediate benefits that will motivate you to WANT to make healthy lifestyle changes that last.

The old saying - we eat because we're happy and we eat because we're sad - certainly applies here.

This whole cycle is illustrated in the diagram below.

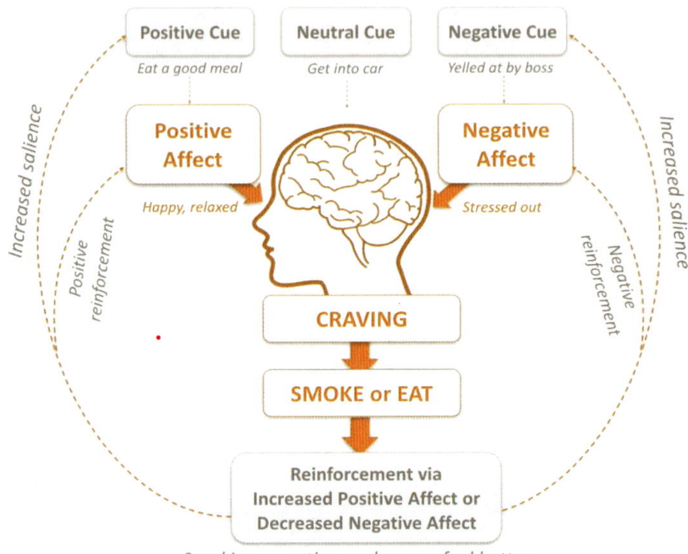

Thorndike 1898, Skinner, 1938, Zinser 1992, Piasecki 1997, Carter 1999, Lazev 1999, Cox 2001, Robinson 2003, Bevins 2004, Baker 2004, Cook 2004, Olausson 2004, Shiffman 2004, Carter 2008, Perkins 2010

This is a powerful loop that isn't easy to break. Most behavioral change specialists from James Prochaska to Stanford psychologist BJ Fogg, have come up with entirely different approaches for interrupting this cycle. BJ Fogg says it's easier to substitute a new habit loop than break an old one. When you feel like smoking a cigarette at lunch, go for a walk instead.

In his best-selling book THE POWER OF HABIT, Charles Duhigg focuses on figuring out exactly what's cueing your behavior. When trying to keep himself from snacking at work in the afternoon he first tries to figure out if it is hunger, boredom or feeling sad that is driving his urge to snack. If it's hunger, he eats a healthy snack, like an apple. If it's boredom, he finds a friend at the water fountain to chat with, if it's feeling sad, he looks to make a quick phone call, or check out an internet meme to cheer himself up. His method for breaking the habit loop is all about deciphering the exact cue.[6]

But Brewer's mindfulness approach is entirely different. He tries to break the habit loop by decoupling craving and behavior. "Whatever strategy we've learned for dealing with a stressful trigger, whether it's eating a cookie, going on Facebook, having a drink, or smoking a cigarette, all these rewards have consequences." Psychologists call this counter-productive coping because these short-term rewards can eventually lead to long-term consequences.

As author and wellness expert Dr. David Katz likes to say: "If you think coping with stress is difficult, try coping with a stress-related dis-ease brought on by your counter-productive coping strategies like eating or smoking whenever you feel stressed."[7] That's what happens when we don't figure out a healthy way to break a bad habit loop.

The gym where I work out, five days a week, (when there's no pandemic) is located right next door to a fast food place. Every time I leave that gym and walk to my car all I can smell is that fast food. In the morning, the air smells like pancakes, and in the afternoon, it smells like French fries.

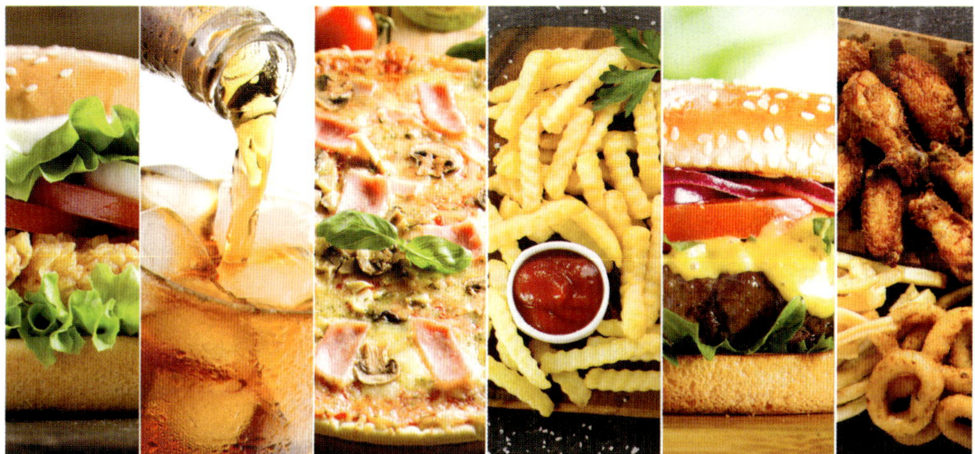

That smell could be a cue or a trigger. I used to eat at that fast food place all the time. Twenty years ago, these smells would have drawn me right in for breakfast or lunch. Now, the smell of their pancakes doesn't trigger me at all. Why? Because I know I will get that fake syrup with my pancakes that I really don't like. So, resisting that cue is easy. But can you see how mindfulness (of what goes *with* the pancakes) drives my decision-making and consequently my behavior?

The smell of French fries in the afternoon is a lot harder to resist. In my youth, that smell was reason enough to pull into a fast food place on a whim. Now, however I know there are better places to get *really good* French fries. I consider that fact very carefully as I walk to my car. Plus, I mindfully consider this additional drawback about this particular brand of fast food – if the fries have been sitting in that metal bin under those heat lamps for too long – they basically turn to little hard sticks of wood. I remind myself: *I don't like eating little hard sticks of wood.* Now you can really see how mindfulness interrupts that craving, too.

Consider this one very important fact: All my ability to resist these cravings came NOT from avoiding them all together. NO, it came from *going* to this place, trying these treats and letting my awareness about THE ACTUAL EXPERIENCE, guide my decision-making. There's really something liberating about this mindfulness strategy.

Here's one last thought about leaving the gym. As Stanford University health psychologist Kelly McGonigle reports in her book entitled The Willpower Instinct "*things that require will power, give you will power.*"[9] When I walk out of that gym feeling great, I have inherently more will power than when I walked in. It took willpower to go to the gym and do that workout. That investment in willpower pays me right back when I leave, every day. In that feel-good, willpower-enhanced state, it's easier to pass on fast food.

A little over a year ago, after leaving the gym I went to the fast food place next door for lunch. Wait, what? Yes, I went to the very same place I said I could easily resist for lunch and I wasn't even that hungry.

Here's what happened. I got into my car after leaving the gym and it wouldn't start. I called emergency roadside assistance and they told me it would take at least an hour, probably two, to respond. While waiting for the tow-truck to arrive I decided to go next door and eat.

So, it wasn't the smell or hunger that was the cue. It was a different cue. It was a combination of annoyance and boredom. It was more of an emotional cue and that pushed me over the edge. Knowing full well that this is NOT how I usually feel after leaving the gym, I KNEW I could go to this fast food place and NOT have to worry one bit about reigniting an old trigger that would start me wanting this brand of fast food again.

I hadn't been to this chain in years, so I decided to do it mindfully. I saw that they had these new gourmet burgers on the menu, so I decided to give one a try. I ordered the meal and I got the fries along with it. I zeroed in on every sensation: I noticed that the bun tasted a little stale, the sauce wasn't quite as tasty as it was at other gourmet burger places, the fries were a little hard, and the Coke (I swear they mess with the formula at this chain) tasted dry like it had too much soda and not enough syrup. So, eating my food mindfully, also helped me to NOT rekindle my old fast food habit loop.

Judson Brewer, M.D., has developed a smart phone app to help people interrupt their habit loops for smoking and eating. The app directs users who are encountering a cue to ride it out using a method he calls R.A.I.N.[10] RAIN is an acronym that stands for:

Recognize: Relax into the knowledge of the craving.

Accept/Allow: It's OK that you are having this craving (don't berate yourself for it, don't judge it.)

Investigate: What exactly is going on? Be curious about it. Curiosity feels good.

Note: What is happening inside your body? What's your cue? Is it pain? Hunger? Sadness? How exactly does it manifest itself in your body?

Since the very first chapter you've seen how mindfulness is about awareness and acceptance. That's all conveniently (mnemonically) spelled out in the RAIN acronym. The R in rain is about awareness. Fully Recognizing the problem and not sweeping it under the rug. The A is all about Acceptance. We are all human, and sometimes the littlest things can trigger a behavioral sequence that's very hard to stop, from having a smoke when we are in a place that other people smoke, to having a warm glazed donut when you see the hot light is on at Krispy Kreme Donuts. Learn to recognize (and be mindful of) the specific cues that trigger the habit loop.

The I is all about going toward the pain and suffering (even if it's minor) instead of backing away from it. Investigate the cue, and the thoughts that the cue triggers. Be curious about WHY you need to have a donut right this minute? And when you Note what's happening inside your body, you may see that there are other options available to you for interrupting this temporary state of craving from simply waiting another 15 minutes before indulging (and often times that's enough to break the cycle) to choosing another behavior entirely, like calling an old friend or going for a walk instead.

Once you have a healthy habit loop in place like working out at the gym, or meditating for five minutes when you come home from work, or going for a walk at lunch, or getting up and stretching for a few minutes every hour during your day, the healthy habits build on themselves and reinforce other healthy habits that do battle with your *unhealthy* habit loops. If I'm feeling great in the morning after a workout, I certainly don't want to ruin that feeling by eating a high fat, high carb fast food breakfast – that I know – will only make me feel tired an hour later.

After my morning workout, my body's feel-good chemicals are just starting to kick in. I feel relaxed because I've exercised away my stress and tension. I feel energized because my body has received the movement it craves. My willpower is strong because what required will power – going to the gym in the first place – is now giving me even more willpower back: the power to resist the tasty smells coming from the building next door.

I haven't been back to that fast food restaurant since that one time, over a year ago.

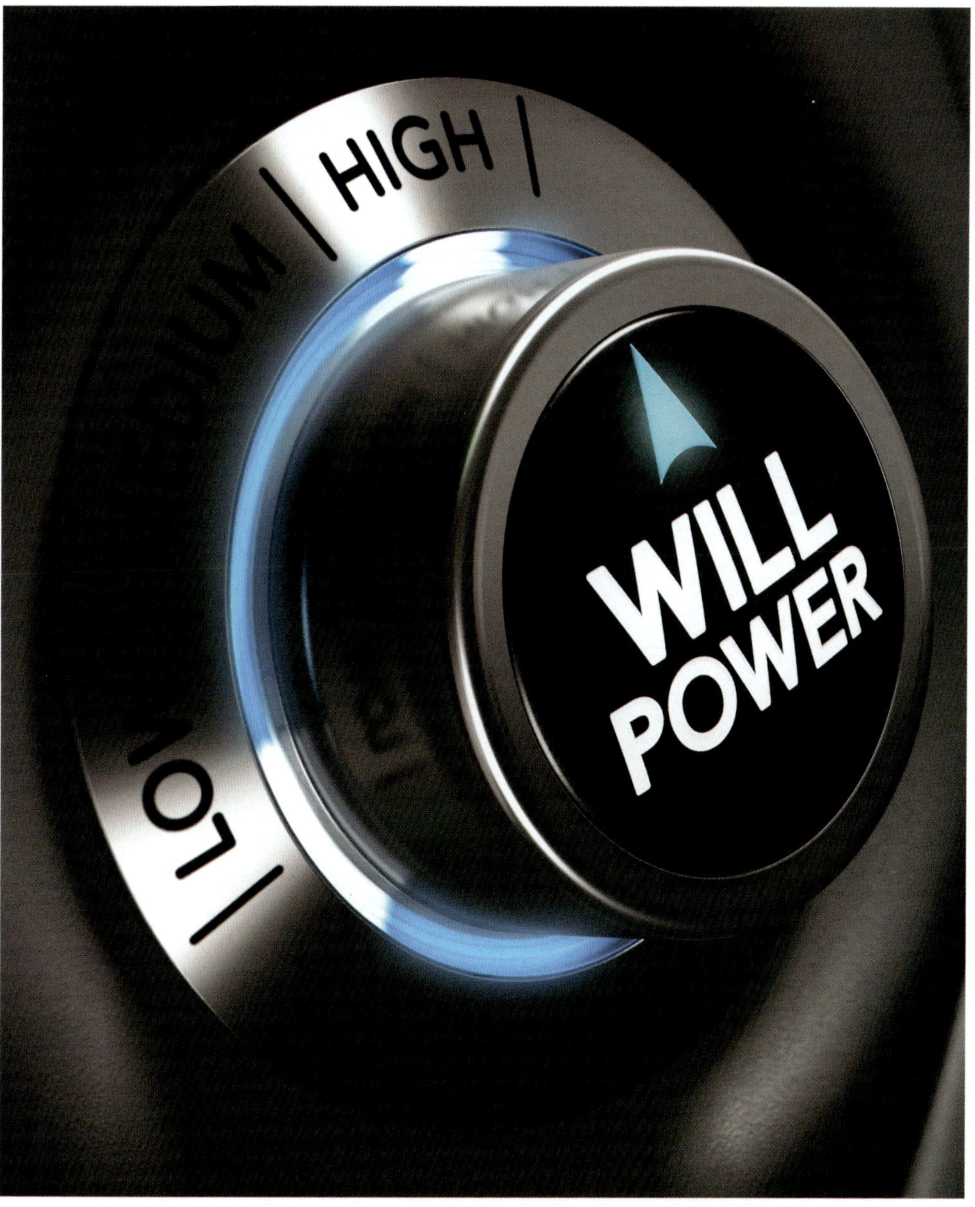

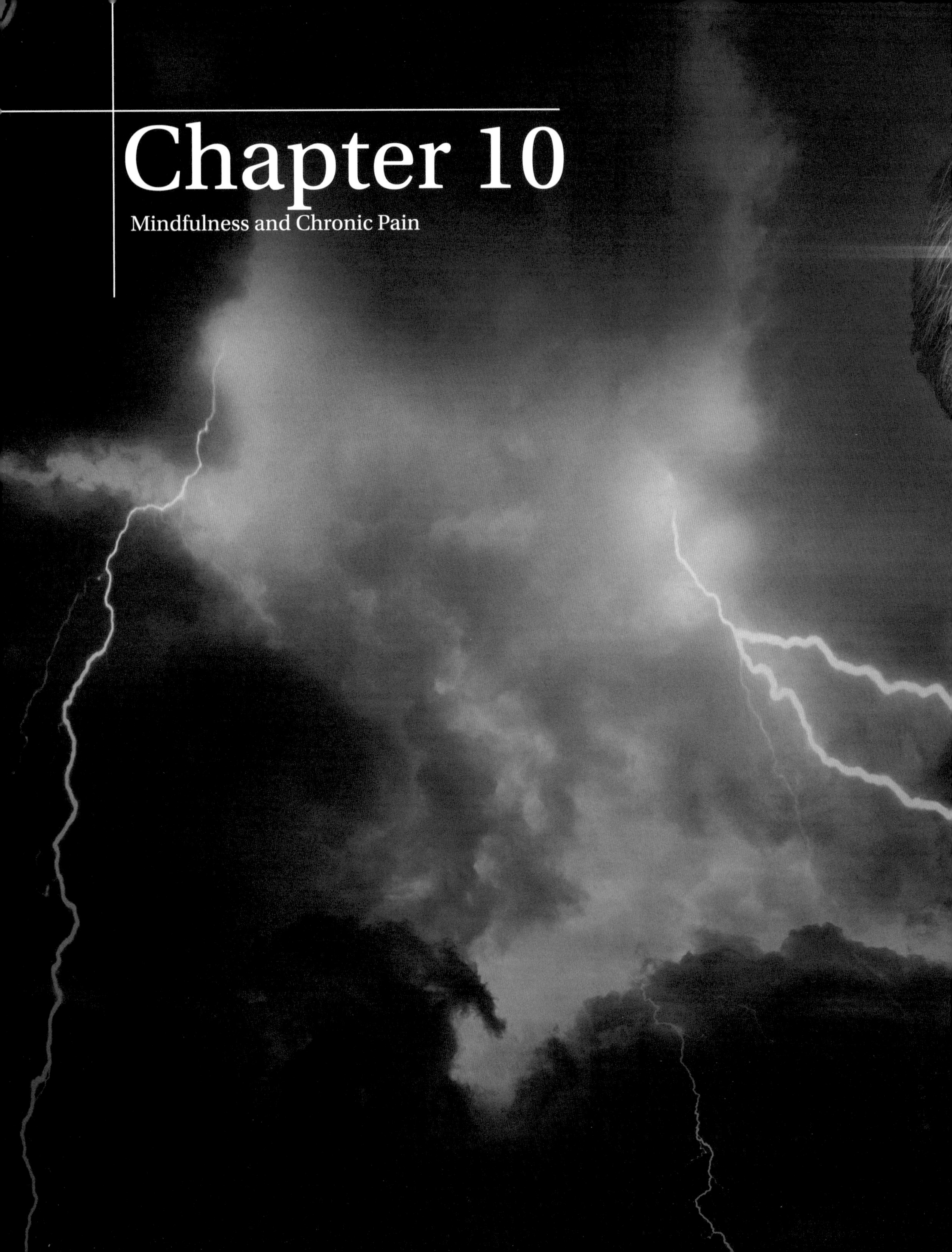

Chapter 10

Mindfulness and Chronic Pain

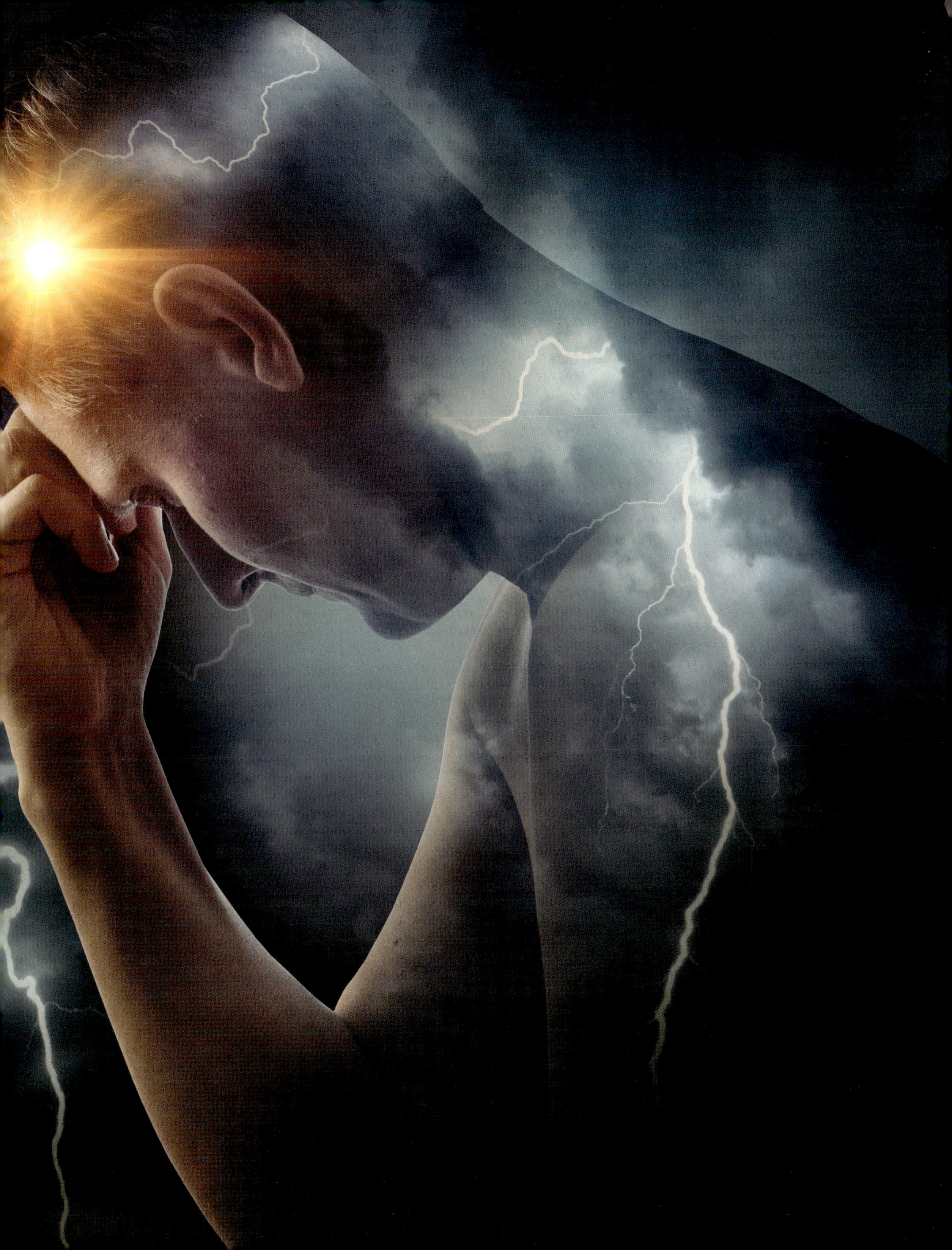

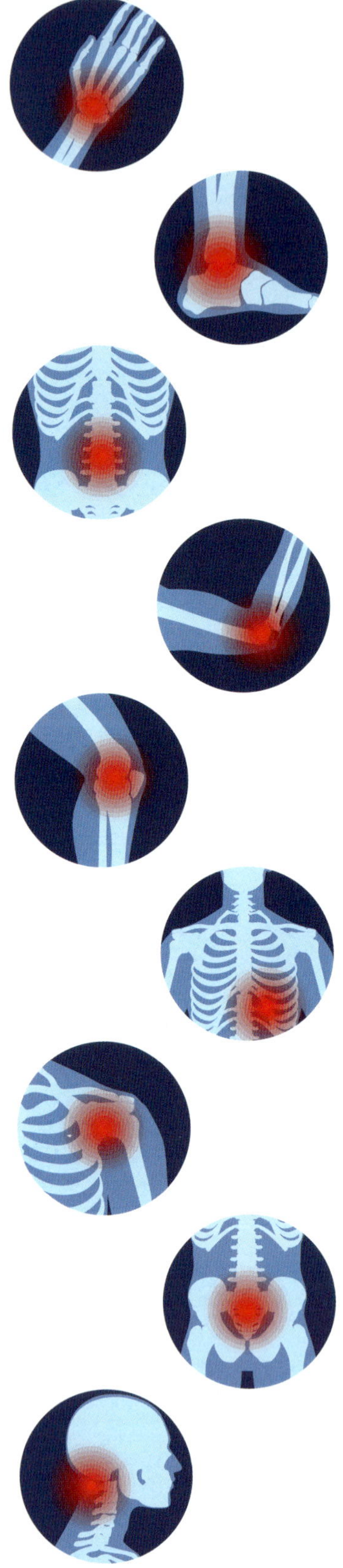

Chapter 10
Mindfulness and Chronic Pain
The Story of Two Arrows

Long before Jon Kabat-Zinn created the very first MBSR course at the University of Massachusetts Medical Center, he attended a two-week retreat during a very cold April month at an abandoned summer camp in the Berkshires Mountains of Western Massachusetts. That retreat was conducted by a Zen meditation teacher named Robert Hover. Mindfulness retreats are often inexpensive, bare-bones affairs with little or no creature comforts to distract one from the real goal of the meditation: *giving it your undivided attention!*

One of the practices that was taught during the two-week retreat was extreme, even for a bare-bones retreat: To sit in meditation for two hours straight, *without moving a muscle.* Jon Kabat-Zinn apparently experienced a kind of back-breaking pain that he described as being some of the worst pain he'd ever experienced in his entire life.[1]

The point of the practice was to try and separate the sensation of pain from *the story about the pain.* Even though the pain was intense, with the standard mindfulness approach of carefully observing this pain, he was able to not only bear it, *but make it disappear.* By continually scanning his body from head to toe, during the two hours of sitting perfectly still, cultivating an awareness below the level of thought, eventually "the pain dissolved into pure sensations."[2]

Already working at the University of Massachusetts Medical Center on a fellowship to study cell biology, Jon Kabat-Zinn thought this method of observing and then reducing pain in meditation, might be a way to help the chronic pain patients at the Medical Center. Many of these patients were dependent on narcotics for controlling their pain. If he could teach them what he had learned during his retreat – in familiar ways that didn't feel threatening to them - maybe that could provide a non-pharmaceutical option for reducing pain. That's how the standardized 8-week MBSR course at the University of Massachusetts Medical Center was born.

One of the things that's hard for almost anyone to understand is that pain – even though it emanates from different places in (or on) our bodies, is entirely manifested in the brain. So, when we take medicine to relieve pain, unless it's a topical cream, it's not going to the place where the pain is coming from, but to the receptors in the brain where that pain is registering. Understanding this important point helps us also understand how mindfulness might work with the brain's *perception of the pain*, and not necessarily at the site of the pain itself.

I have learned a trick for how to shut down the low-level pain of itching. While this little trick isn't going to help you with chronic pain, it WILL help you understand how the pain receptors in your brain work. Minor pain, like itching, uses the same neural pathways between the surface of your skin and the brain as do more intense forms of pain such as a cut or a burn you might get in the very same spot. But the more intense pain, always takes priority on this shared neural pathway, *whenever the two forms of pain overlap.* When the intense pain is over, your brain flips a switch on this pain receptor to off and doesn't register any minor pain coming from the same spot for the next couple of hours.[3]

Here's my trick for stopping the itch. I soak the itchy spot on my skin under warm running water in the sink (if it's on my arms), or from a removable shower head in the bath tub (if the itch is on my leg, for example). I gradually turn up the heat on the running water. When I get *just* past my own pain threshold but long before there would be any kind of burn, I shut the water off. My brain gets the signal from the nerve (connected to the itch) that the intense (burning) pain is over, and it flips the receptor off. Since ALL itches are made worse by scratching, sometimes the two-hour break I get from itching, is enough to actually CURE it.

Not only does this hot water trick give you a great method for getting rid of an annoying itch, it helps you understand how the PERCEPTION of pain takes place in the brain. And if you can fool the brain into not perceiving pain in this way, maybe there are other ways you can fool it, too. And this leads to the next most important thing I've ever learned about mindfulness: *The Story of the Two Arrows.*

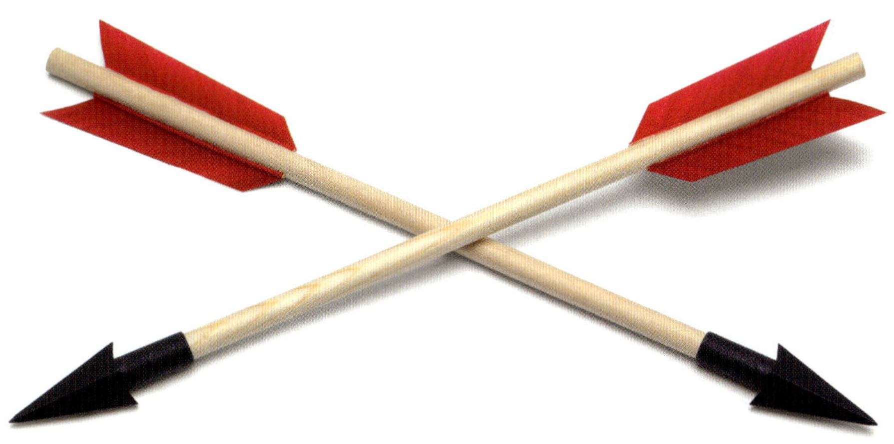

I learned this mindfulness story from Dr. Ron Siegel, the professor at Harvard who taught me about state and trait effects. I love this tale because it helps you understand the psychology of pain in a way that also helps you learn how to manage it.

The first arrow represents the real pain we feel when we get physically hurt. We ALL get struck by arrows, whether it's a muscle pull, a migraine headache, a back spasm, a stomachache, or an injury that requires medical care. Unfortunately, pain, injury and sickness are a very real part of living. *That's the first arrow.*

The second arrow represents the story you tell yourself ABOUT the pain: Why me? Why do I have to deal with this pain? This pain is terrible. It's constant. I wouldn't have this pain right now if that so and so hadn't run into my car at 70 miles per hour. *We've all been struck by this second arrow, too.*

Mindfulness helps us separate the real physical pain of the first arrow from the psychological pain of the second arrow. That's apparently what Jon Kabat-Zinn did in his two-hour meditation. This understanding of how pain works on both a physical and psychological level, can significantly increase your pain threshold because you are *perceiving* less pain overall.

Secondary Stress Response

Whenever you feel stressed, there's always the chance that you will experience a secondary stress response, right after the first one. Maybe you've had the experience of waking up in the middle of the night feeling anxious. It's hard to fall back to sleep when you're anxious. The more anxious you become the more awake you get. As a result, you feel stressed about being stressed. This is a classic example of a secondary stress response.

A secondary stress response is similar to the story of the two arrows: We experience pain, and then there's the pain we feel about feeling pain: Why does this happen to me? Or, when we feel embarrassed, we start to blush; somebody points that out, and suddenly we're embarrassed about being embarrassed.

Mindfulness practice is all about watching your pain, your worry, your stress and your embarrassment and not reacting to it. Just letting it be. So, it just sits there and doesn't multiply. It never gets to this secondary level of stress. While this takes practice, it's enormously liberating when you master your ability to let your problem be exactly what it is. When you learn to objectively monitor your pain, you will be surprised to see how often, you can minimize it and sometimes, make it disappear entirely.

The amazing thing about mindfulness is you don't even have to convince yourself that the second arrow isn't just as consequential as the first. All you need do is OBSERVE the actual (physical) pain and then *notice* how it is separate from the psychological pain. *It's all about cultivating awareness.*

When it comes to chronic pain, being in the present moment means acknowledging the pain when it's there – but also acknowledging the times when it's NOT there. And more importantly, acknowledging the fact that this pain will most likely fluctuate. Everything in life is in a state of flux. (This is the same concept as impermanence which we discussed in chapter 4). When we are experiencing good times – these good times will change. But when we are experiencing bad times – including pain – that is most likely going to change (come and go) too.

Talking about stress, Elissa Epel, a psychologist at the University of California, San Francisco said: "One thing to remember about chronic stress is that it's only our thoughts that make it seem so. Viewed mindfully, no situation is truly chronic — there are always calm moments to notice and be present for. Moments that can be lived in with ease."[4] The same idea can be applied to pain.

V.S. Ramachandran is a world-famous neuroscientist, author and professor at the University of California, San Diego. Dr. Ramachandran has developed a unique approach for treating veterans who served in Iraq and Afghanistan and who suffer from a rare form of chronic pain known as phantom limb syndrome.

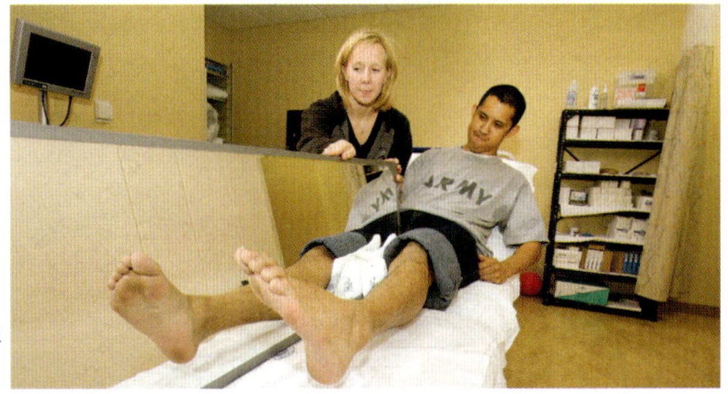

Patients with phantom limb syndrome often still feel pain (and sometimes it's excruciating pain) in limbs that have long since been amputated. "My missing limb feels paralyzed and if I could move it, it might help me alleviate the pain," one patient told Dr. Ramachandran. In his book, THE TELL-TALE BRAIN, the doctor writes that, often times, a person whose limbs are amputated, will have suffered with a painful, fractured, dysfunctional version of that same limb for months, before it is finally severed.

> "Imagine during a long period of convalescence, (after the initial injury but before the amputation) pain shoots through his hand every time he moves it. His brain is seeing a constant 'If A then B' pattern where A is movement and B is pain. Thus, the synapses between the neurons that represent these two events are strengthened daily, for months on end. Eventually the very attempt to move the hand elicits excruciating pain."[5]

Ramachandran then wondered if there was a way for his patients to somehow "see" their missing arm and move it, would they be able to fool the brain and alleviate the pain that was mysteriously locked there? Ramachandran then rigged up a special box with a mirror inside that would allow the patient to "see" the missing arm. When the patient inserts his intact arm into the box and looks in the mirror, *he sees what looks like his missing arm.* As far as his brain is concerned this is the missing arm. By being able to move it, this movement greatly reduced or eliminated the pain of the imagined paralysis.

Ramachandran set up one more version of this experiment, where he asked the patient with phantom limb syndrome to look at the mirror image of the intact arm through a minimizing lens (the opposite of a magnifying glass). The patient was shocked. Ramachandran writes that his patient exclaimed: "My phantom not only looks small but feels small as well. The pain has shrunk too. Down to about one fourth of the intensity it was before."[6]

And that's what Jon Kabat-Zinn – in a completely different way - taught the pain patients at his clinic: How to see their pain through the minimizing lens of mindfulness. By first identifying and greatly reducing the story around the pain – the second arrow – that psychological distance would minimize the overall levels of pain significantly.

As Jon Kabat-Zinn writes in his first book, Full Catastrophe Living, when the pain clinic at the hospital would send over patients to The Stress Reduction Clinic, the patients who just wanted their doctor to make the pain go away were NOT the best candidates for this mindfulness approach. Usually these patients wanted a quick fix, i.e., a pill.

But for many others the slow-going mindfulness approach worked exceedingly well. These were the patients who, after multiple surgeries and various medications, *would still be suffering from chronic pain.* At that point they were told by their doctors: "You just have to learn to live with the pain." But as Jon Kabat-Zinn writes: "They were never taught how. Being told that you have to live with the pain should not be the end of the road but the beginning."[7]

As an MIT-trained scientist, Jon Kabat-Zinn wanted proof that his approach to treating pain patients worked. He conducted various studies right from the beginning that he writes about in his book. "In one study 61 percent of the patients with chronic pain achieved at least a 50 percent reduction in pain. This improvement was accompanied by a sharp drop (55 percent) in negative mood states, an increase in positive mood states, and major improvements in anxiety, depression, and hostility."[8]

He and his team also compared two groups of 21 patients (42 total), each going to the hospital pain clinic over a ten-week period. One of the two groups split off and also took the 8-week mindfulness course at the Stress Reduction Clinic. The first group, who didn't participate in the meditation, "showed little change over the ten weeks." While the meditating group experienced "major improvements."[9]

This was one of the very first scientific studies proving the benefits of mindfulness. Now there are thousands of studies, printed in medical and psychological journals, published around the world, that confirm what Jon Kabat-Zinn had suspected long ago at a cold, bare-bones retreat center in the Berkshire mountains of western Massachusetts.

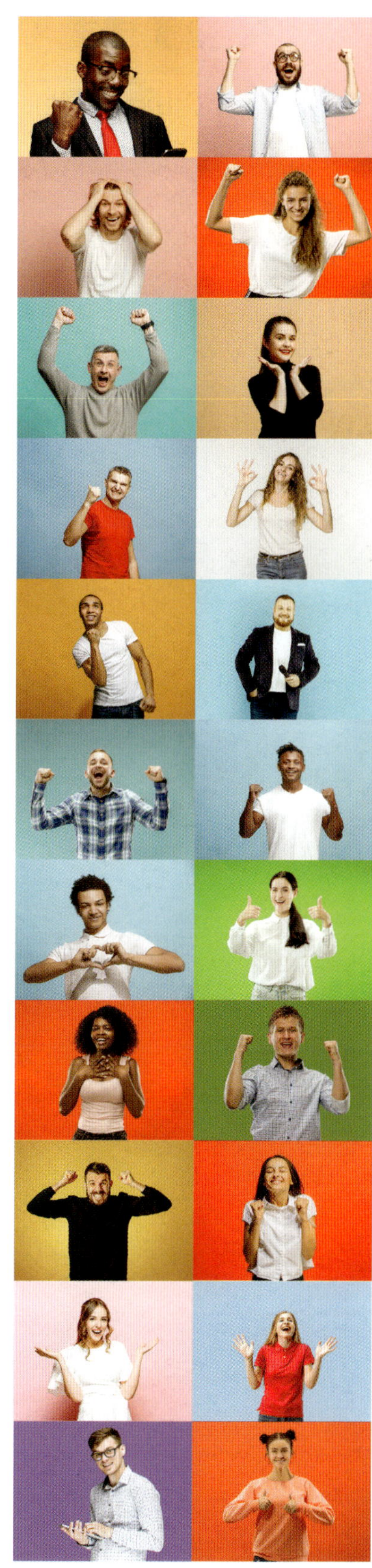

Chapter 11

Mindfulness and Acceptance

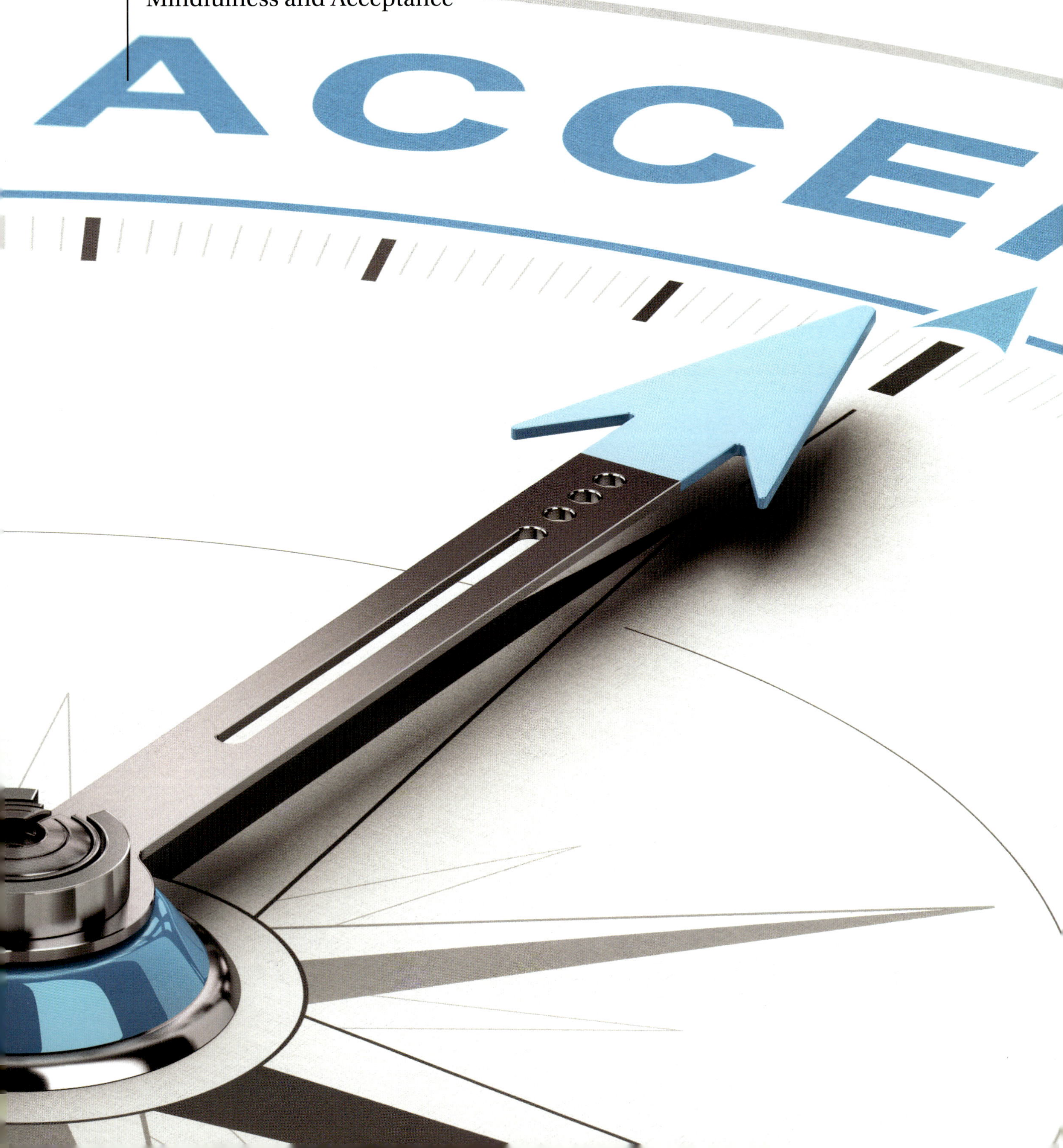

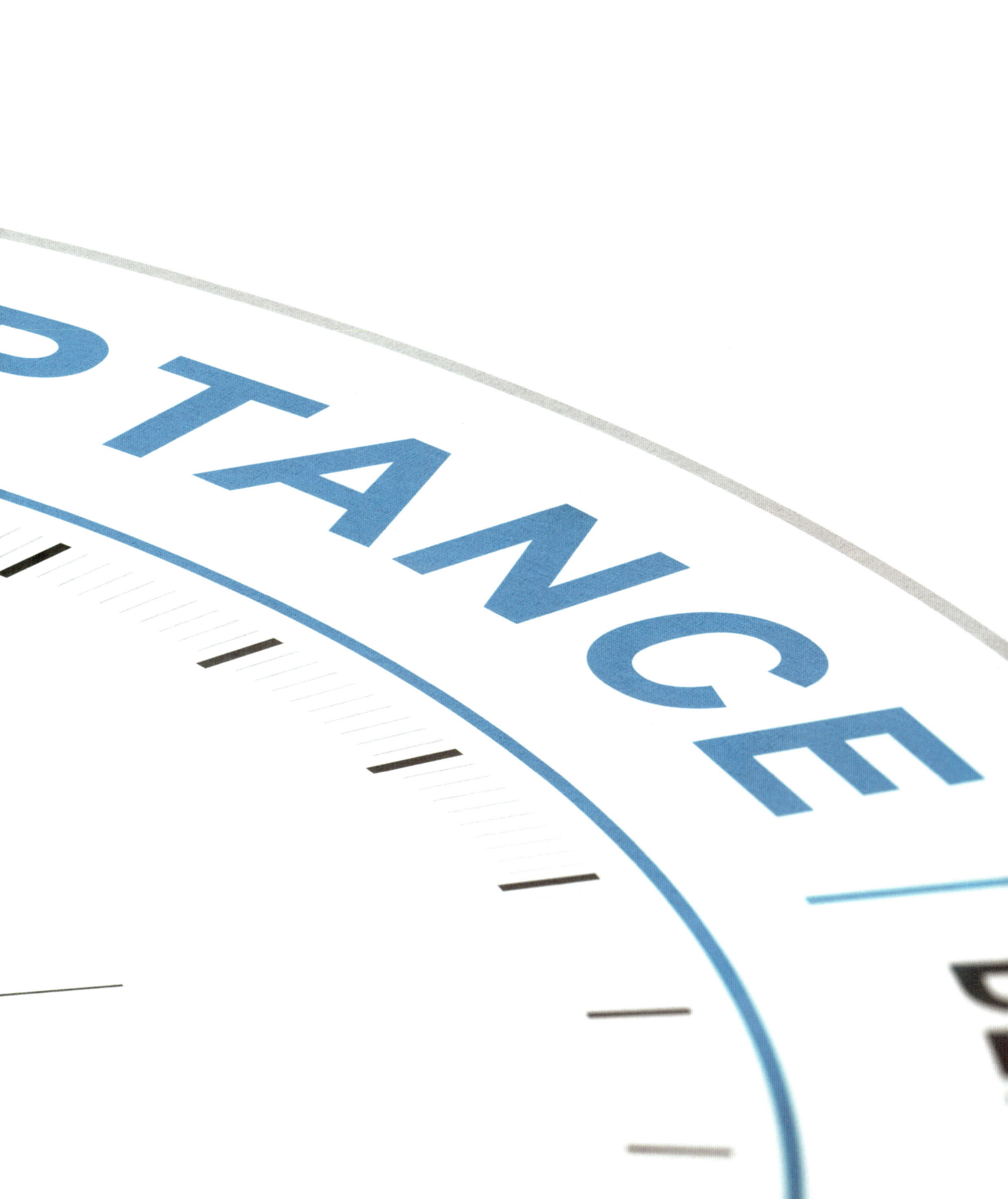
TANCE

Chapter 11
Mindfulness and Acceptance

Most people seem to know that mindfulness has something to do with being in the present moment. What barely anyone knows is that you can't even BE in the present moment without acceptance. Author and mindfulness expert Dr. Ron Siegel defines mindfulness as "*present moment awareness with acceptance.*"

It's a good definition, because in order to *truly* be in the present moment you must accept whatever the present moment brings. While the present moment can be wonderful and easy to embrace when you're gazing up at the stars at night, looking at a beautiful sunset, or lying on a warm beach, it can be quite difficult to embrace when you're stuck in traffic, listening to noisy neighbors, dealing with annoying coworkers or worried about something much more serious like a pandemic.

How are you supposed to be "in the moment" then?

That's where acceptance comes in. Acceptance of the present moment encompasses everything that's bothering you in the present moment, *including your inability to accept it*. As you will see, in mindfulness, by taking an additional step back, acceptance can ALWAYS bring some measure of peace no matter what kind of chaos the present moment brings into your life.

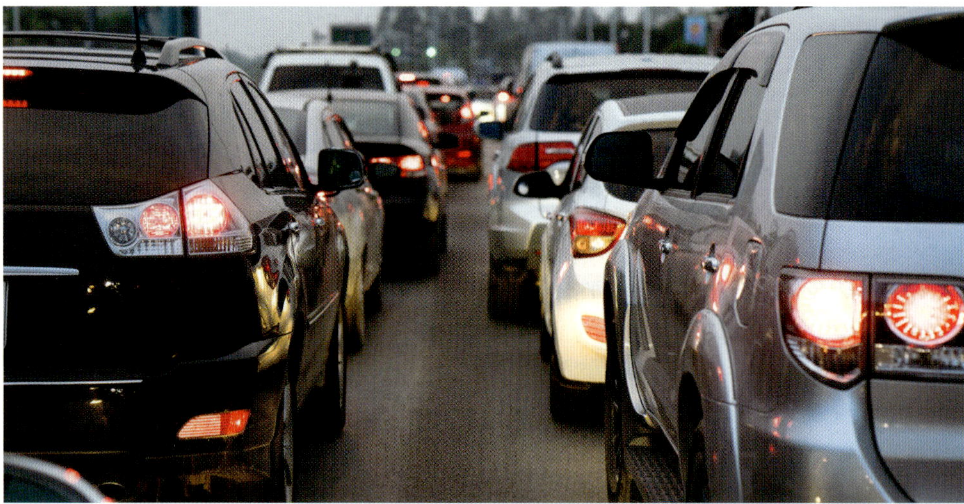

Let's say, you're stuck in traffic. You've tried saying, "Hey it's just a traffic jam, what's the big deal!" And that didn't work. You've tried accepting the fact that you are now going to be late for work, and that *really* didn't work. You've even tried taking a couple of deep breaths but that didn't work either. You're just plain annoyed, or worried or fearful and there's no getting over it. What do you do?

Accept the fact that you can't accept it.

This may sound crazy but hear me out. Instead of sweeping your negative emotions, your worries, your fear, your anger or your annoyance under the rug and trying to pretend like it's not there, this approach says that it's OK to be annoyed; It's OK to be angry;

It's OK to be frustrated; It's OK to be worried, if you just accept it. This extra measure of acceptance puts a little space around your emotions, and sometimes, it's just enough space, that the difficult moment either becomes bearable, or possibly even recedes into the background.

This acceptance might come in the form of noticing your annoyance and saying to yourself: *Wow, look at how annoyed I am over this traffic jam; Wow, look at how worried I am about this possible health scare.* (Remember the skill we taught in chapter 4 called name it and tame it? That's what we are talking about here.) Simply observing how you feel can bring you back into the present moment with acceptance.

Maybe the most important lesson I ever learned about acceptance was something I had to accept about myself. Something that at first seemed like a character flaw. Many years ago, I was asked to speak to a support group for adults with ADD. I knew very little about ADD at the time. When I arrived at the place where I was to present, there was a flyer on a table by the door entitled, 11 Signs and Symptoms of ADD. I read through the list and I realized I had 10 out of the 11 signs.

Initially this was hard to accept. I really didn't like the fact that I had a mental health problem that actually had a name! But that name explained why I easily misplace things, why I lose things, why I'm disorganized, why I forget the names of people I've just met, and why I tend to run late for meetings. Eventually it was a relief to know exactly what was wrong with me. This was the beginning of my road to acceptance.

That's when I started reading books about ADD and learning all kinds of strategies to keep myself from losing things and forgetting people's names and staying organized and getting places on time. Now I rarely forget things anymore, but when I do, I don't get frustrated or down on myself because I accept the fact that this is who I AM! I do whatever I have to do to move on and/or correct the problem at whatever cost. There's just no point in getting upset about it because that would mean I only accept the part of me that I LIKE. No, I must accept ALL of me or this acceptance trick doesn't work.

BUT, if I notice that I AM having ANY trouble accepting any of the above, *I accept the fact I can't accept it.* And that's the amazing thing about mindfulness. It is infinitely flexible in this way. You can ALWAYS take one step back from where you are standing (especially when you feel stuck or down on yourself for making a mistake) and find a place of acceptance that puts you back in this moment right here and right now: Whether that's *accepting* that you have a noisy neighbor, or *accepting* that you're too timid to speak up to this noisy neighbor or *accepting* (or realizing) that you can be a noisy neighbor too, there's lots of room for you to step back (and gain perspective) when it comes to mindful acceptance.

When my daughter turned 13, I took her and two of her friends into New York City to see a matinee performance of a Broadway show for her birthday. We got into the TKTS line in Times Square, where you can buy half-price tickets on the day of the show. When we got near the front of the line, there was a video terminal that displayed all the shows that still had tickets left for that day. Some days you have a lot more choices than on other days. Luckily, this was one of those days when there were a lot of choices.

I told my daughter she could pick out any show. I noticed that the musical Hairspray was one of the options. I had taken our whole family to see that show about a month earlier and we just watched the movie version of it the previous night, so I was hoping she

Mindfulness at the Movies

Mindful acceptance requires you to stay in the present moment. It's when you fail to notice that your mind has taken you someplace far away, that you lose the present moment. Sometimes this mind-wandering is almost like a movie playing out in your head.

These movies, often staring "poor me," have so much impact, you feel like you are sitting in the front row at an IMAX movie. Even though your story may be complete fiction, it feels 100% real. These little dramatizations can have an effect on your mood, making it even more difficult to accept what it is you are worrying about or getting yourself upset about.

So, when you find yourself in the middle of one of these mental IMAX movies, and you want to reach a place of acceptance, imagine the screen is far away, like a drive-in movie you were watching outside the parking lot from across the street. The farther away you are from the screen the more aware of the present moment you become. The story starts to lose its hold over you.

Maybe you are replaying an embarrassing moment from your past on your personal IMAX screen. Step as far back as you can to gain awareness. Awareness of the present moment tells you: this "poor me" story happened two weeks ago. Acceptance says: Nobody even remembers it or even cares.

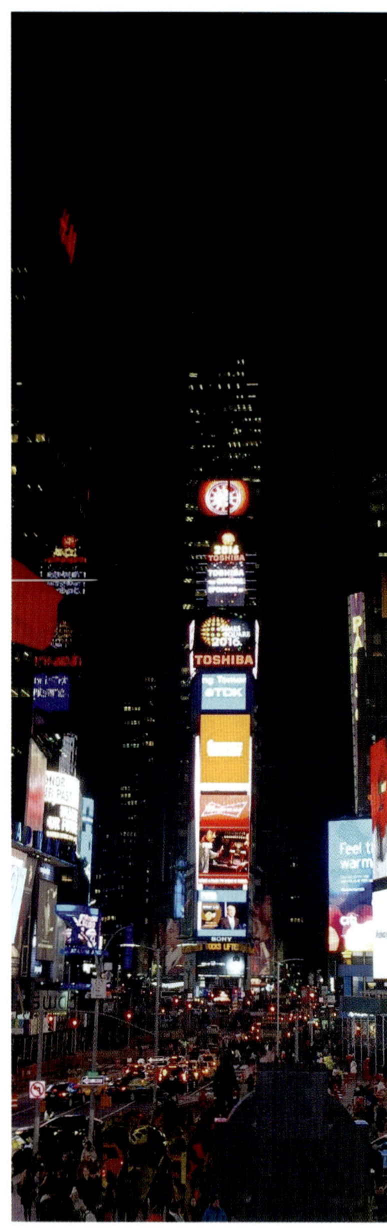

wouldn't pick that musical because we'd already seen it AND I really didn't like it all that much. A minute later she asked: "Is it OK if we see Hairspray again Dad?"

On some level, I wanted to say: Couldn't you pick another show we haven't already seen - *twice*? But instead I said, "OK." I got out my credit card and paid over $300 to buy four *half-priced* tickets to see a show I didn't even like. For the next ten minutes or so I was sulking and beating myself up, for not making her pick another show. Now as you can see, this story has suddenly become a "poor me" story and not at all about my daughter. (Remember what we said about I, ME and MINE in chapter 4?)

Ego plays a big role in events which we have difficulty accepting. Our ego says things like: I shouldn't have to wait in a long line. Children should be well-behaved. People should always treat me with respect. And, in this case, I shouldn't have to pay $300 to see a show I've already seen and didn't even like.

Psychologist Albert Ellis writes about how we all need to break away from the irrational notion that: "Things upset me," and move on to the more truthful notion that "I upset myself." And a lot of the time it's ego, rearing its ugly head that upsets us, and makes it difficult to accept the situation and move on.

So, I'm standing in a souvenir store a few minutes later, holding 4 tickets to Hairspray and listening to the devil (my ego) on one shoulder saying: "Why didn't I just tell her to pick another show?" And then the angel on the other shoulder is saying: "But it's HER birthday. You told her she could pick ANY show." This battle was going on inside my head as my daughter and her friends were laughing and joking and picking out souvenirs in the store. *They were delighted to be seeing this show.*

That's when I heard the very practical voice of acceptance (the angel) say: "You've already paid for the tickets. You can't go back and buy other tickets. *Accept what is and can't be changed.*"

"But in order to enjoy yourself," the more accepting inner voice continued, "why don't you focus on their happiness and stop worrying about your own." As it turned out, we were unable to get four seats together, so I wound up sitting by myself in the row right behind them. At first, I was bummed out by this arrangement too, but even this minor setback worked out to my advantage: I was ideally situated to watch them, whispering little comments to each other, giggling and having a great time. I walked out of that show on cloud nine, having had one of the best times at a Broadway show, *ever.*

Mindful acceptance is all about liberation. It frees you from past and present hurts and allows you to be in the moment fully. I could have spent that entire show sitting in a row by myself, sulking. It was acceptance that allowed me to open up to the moment rather than shut it down.

But acceptance of what is and can't be changed does NOT mean you have to just accept *everything* that comes your way. It's important to stand up to unfairness, oppression and injustice. You should certainly NOT accept these and other wrongs that have been thrust upon you by society, your community, your employer or a dysfunctional family. Whether it's an abusive relationship, a toxic boss, human injustice, or a job that conflicts with your deepest values, these untenable situations should NOT be accepted.

But even in these challenging situations, where you must fight the status quo, or what seems like an "*unrightable wrong*," (to quote Don Quixote from the song: The Impossible Dream) there are ways of doing it peacefully, while still bringing about the change you wish to see. Mahatma Gandhi and Martin Luther King showed the whole world just how peaceful practices like non-violence and civil disobedience could help overcome oppression and injustice. Gandhi's famous quote "be the change you want to see in the world," inspires us all to want to do the same.

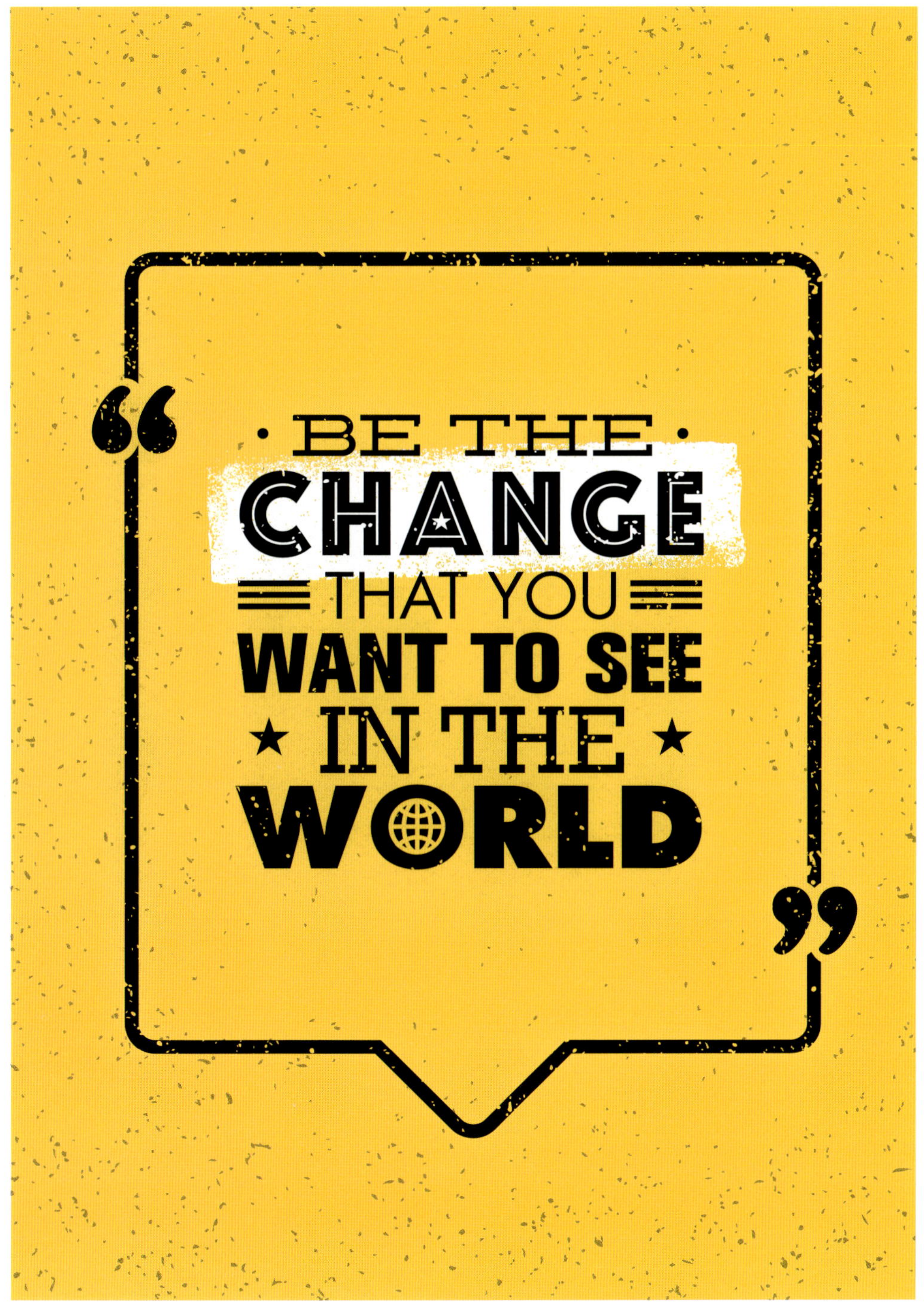

Chapter 12

Mindfulness and Self-actualization

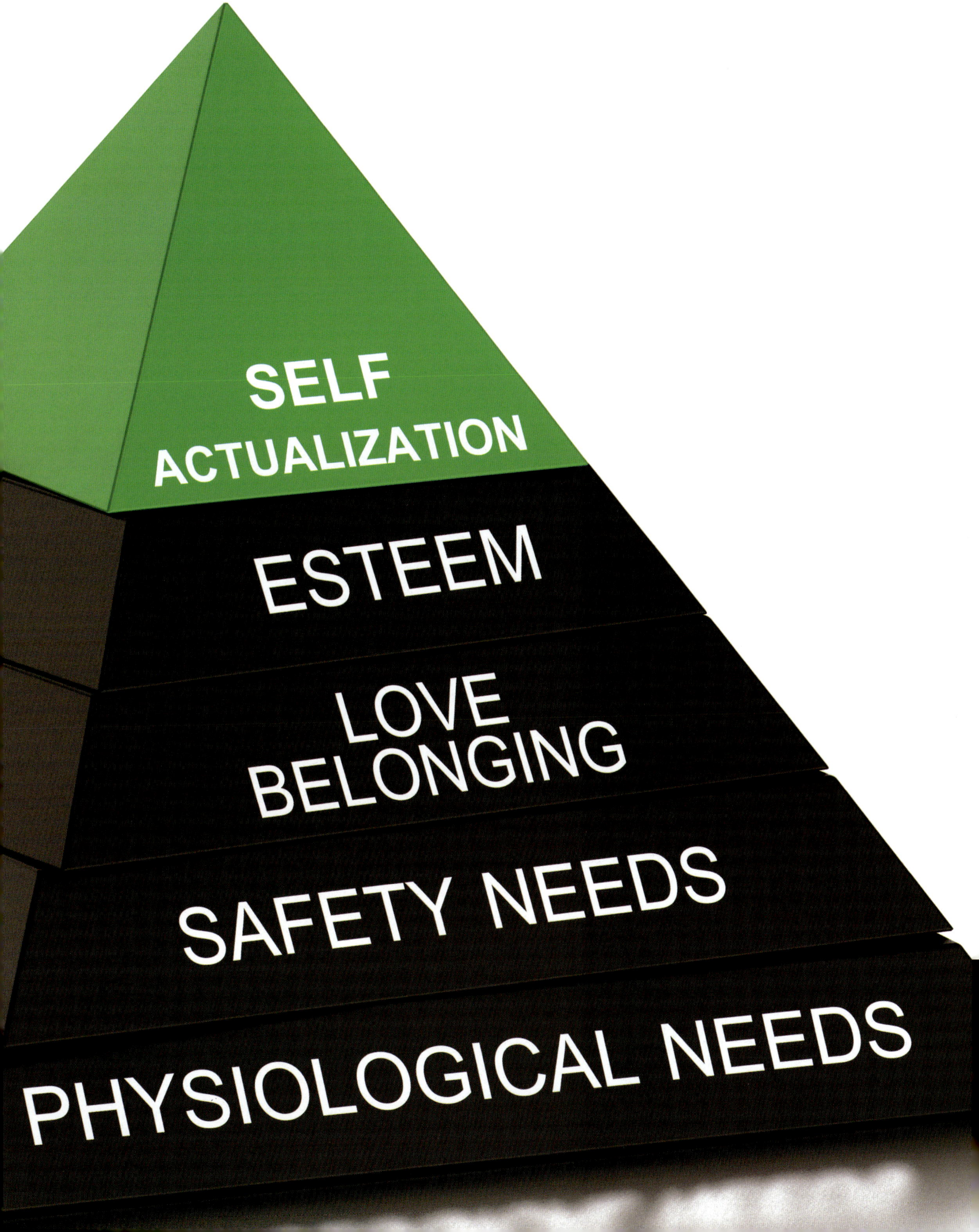

SELF
ACTUALIZATION

ESTEEM

LOVE
BELONGING

SAFETY NEEDS

PHYSIOLOGICAL NEEDS

Chapter 12
Mindfulness and Self-actualization

Of all the people I've ever studied with or worked with, from Albert Ellis to Jon Kabat-Zinn, no one walks his talk quite like Dan Goleman, author of the best-selling books on Emotional Intelligence. He's a pleasure to be around. He is patient, kind, never brags and is a serious mindfulness meditator. He truly is *emotionally intelligent*.

In the 1970's, right out of Harvard, Dan went to India to meet and briefly study meditation with the same meditation teacher – Neem Karoli Baba - whose continuing influence (even after he died) would bring Julia Roberts, Steve Jobs, and even Mark Zuckerberg to India to learn more about him and to study meditation, too.[1]

It seems to me the ONE thing that all these famous sojourners had or have in common, was the desire for self-actualization. And perhaps we can attribute at least some of their success to their fervent desire to fully understand and practice the art of mindfulness.

Certainly not all self-actualized people have studied mindfulness and not all people who study mindfulness become self-actualized. And most importantly, we shouldn't confuse self-actualization with mindfulness, or success for that matter, either. That said, it seems to me, that mindfulness meditation offers every single person who tries it a potential fast track to this lofty goal.

Most of us have trouble getting *out* of our own way. We stumble over self-limiting beliefs that handicap any chance of us truly accomplishing what we want to achieve, either in business or in life or in both. We blame others for our mistakes, we blame the world for being unfair, we blame our bosses for not promoting us, or we blame our parents for not properly raising us. And yet, we hear story after story of people like Oprah Winfrey, or Richard Branson (founder of Virgin Airlines) who pull themselves out of poverty and/or a chaotic childhood to achieve enormous success and true self-actualization.

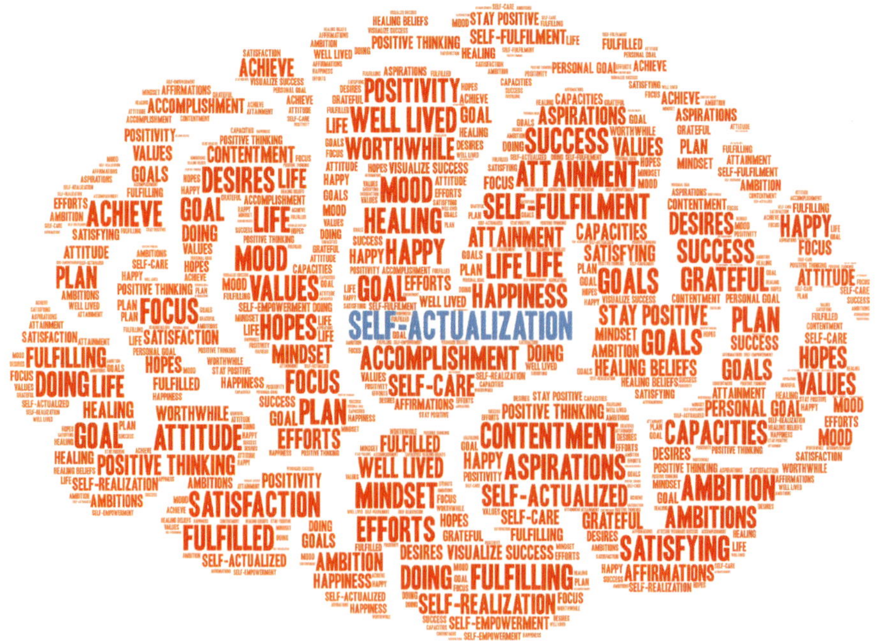

Abraham Maslow, the father of positive (humanistic) psychology, is probably most responsible for popularizing this term: *self-actualization*. He defined it as: "the full realization of one's potential" and of one's "true self."

In searching for the exact qualities of a self-actualized person, I found this list on Wikipedia:[2]

Efficient perceptions of reality. Self-actualizers are able to judge situations correctly and honestly. They are very sensitive to the fake and dishonest and are free to see reality 'as it is'.

Comfortable acceptance of self, others and nature. Self-actualizers accept their own human nature with all its flaws. The shortcomings of others and the contradictions of the human condition are accepted with humor and tolerance.

Reliant on their own experiences and judgement. Independent, not reliant on culture and environment to form their opinions and views.

Spontaneous and natural. True to oneself, rather than being how others want us to be.

Task centering. Most of Maslow's subjects had a mission to fulfill in life or some task or problem 'beyond' themselves to pursue. Humanitarians such as Albert Schweitzer are considered to have possessed this quality. (Jon Kabat-Zinn could certainly be mentioned here too.)

Autonomy. Self-actualizers are free from reliance on external authorities or other people. They tend to be resourceful and independent.

Continued freshness of appreciation. The self-actualizer seems to constantly renew appreciation of life's basic goods. A sunset or a flower will be experienced as intensely time after time as it was at first. There is an "innocence of vision" like that of an artist or a child.

Profound interpersonal relationships. The interpersonal relationships of self-actualizers are marked by deep loving bonds.

Comfort with solitude. Despite their satisfying relationships with others, self-actualizing people value solitude and are comfortable being alone.

Non-hostile sense of humor. This includes the ability to laugh at oneself.

Peak experiences. All of Maslow's subjects reported the frequent occurrence of peak experiences (temporary moments of self-actualization). These occasions were marked by feelings of ecstasy, harmony, and deep meaning. Self-actualizers reported feeling at one with the universe, stronger and calmer than ever before, filled with light, beauty, goodness, and so forth.

It's easy to see the similarities between the qualities of self-actualization and everything I've written about mindfulness up to this point. From acceptance to the "innocence of vision" to comfort with solitude, to peak experiences, there isn't one aspect of self-actualization that isn't an important aspect of mindfulness, also.

If you look at the first three qualities alone, you'll notice something very important about self-actualization that is just as important to mindfulness that we haven't talked about until now: *Perception.*

Ever heard the expression: Perception is reality? The philosophy behind mindfulness says no, *perception is NOT reality.* The fact is, most of us perceive the world through a filter of likes and dislikes, preferences and predilections, memories and past experience, views of the world our parents had (or the exact opposite), and views of the world that are fed to us by our favorite influencers, commentators, news organizations, and radio talk-show hosts. The problem with seeing the world through these different lenses, is that it makes it IMPOSSIBLE for us to see the world as it truly is. We can't even BEGIN to construct reality through these filters.

Deepak Chopra summed up this shortcoming in all human beings when he said: "It's not that we believe what we see, *it's that we see what we already believe.*"[3] When Native Americans first saw Spanish armadas sailing off the coast of America, it's reported that they thought they were seeing tiny floating islands. These floating islands had their own clouds (sails), thunder (cannons), trees (the masts) and landscape (the decks).[4] In other words, we can ONLY see the world through the lens of what WE ALREADY KNOW.

Mindfulness meditation can break this perceptual stranglehold. By emptying out the mind, even for brief (peak experience) moments of meditation, we move our thoughts and perception to a whole new dimension. This can sometimes be an almost sacred place where we are free from the self-limiting beliefs that have prevented us – for our entire lives - from becoming the person WE really *want* to become.

Most of us live in a choiceless world where everything we do is a lockstep version of what we did the day before. When you consider the fact that you probably start each day with the same beverage, eat roughly the same things for breakfast, take the same route to work, sit in all the same places (whether that's your favorite table at a restaurant or your favorite spot on the floor of an exercise class) watch the same types of movies (romcoms, action, horror, or whatever), complain about the same things, and worry or don't worry to the same extent every night, you can see how a lifetime of thoughts and behaviors have led you to where you may be right now. STUCK!

It's very hard to free ourselves from this mass of preprogramming without a LOT of help from an outside, neutral source. *Mindfulness meditation can be that source.*

On a practical level, even when you meditate, you will see that thoughts cross your mind, seemingly from a new place, you never had access to before. These ideas pop in out of leftfield and are brimming with promise, possibility and even practicality. Dan Goleman told me, that when he meditates, he keeps a pad and pencil beside him just in case the next big idea crosses his mind, and he can't wait for the meditation to be over to write it down.

Mindfulness practice provides us with a map for how to get to self-actualization by allowing us to bypass the all too common misperceptions that stop us and so many others. You now have a pretty good idea of what that map might look like: It involves meditating, staying in the present moment, cultivating an awareness below the level of thought, detaching yourself from thoughts and emotions and removing the lenses of preferences, likes and dislikes from your field of vision to see the world as it really is.

Abraham Maslow, however, has a completely different map, and it's usually displayed in the form of the "Hierarchy of Needs" pyramid which you see below:

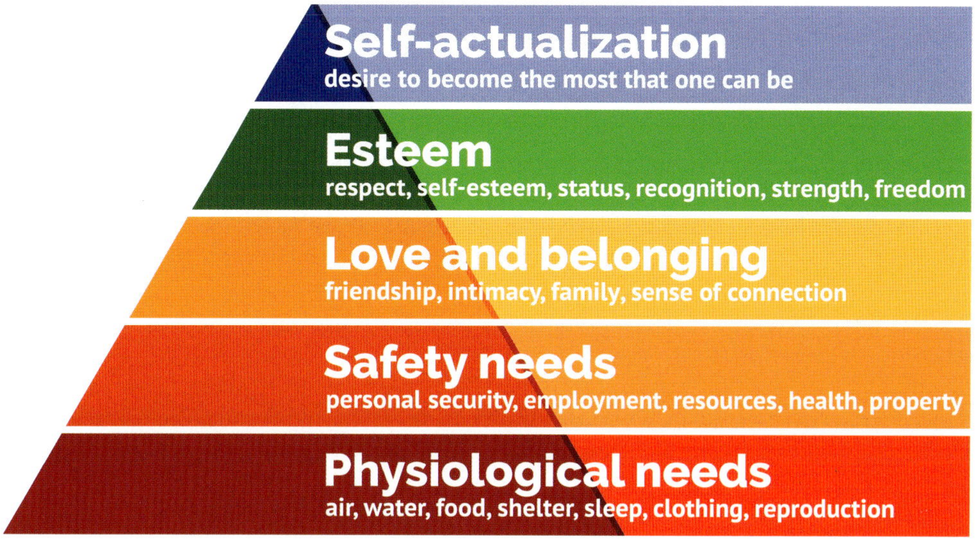

Self-actualization
desire to become the most that one can be

Esteem
respect, self-esteem, status, recognition, strength, freedom

Love and belonging
friendship, intimacy, family, sense of connection

Safety needs
personal security, employment, resources, health, property

Physiological needs
air, water, food, shelter, sleep, clothing, reproduction

In order to get to the point of self-actualization, you have to first attend to certain basic needs. Early interpretations of the pyramid stated that as one's basic needs for food, water, shelter and safety were met, a person moved up the pyramid to meeting one's need for friends, love, belonging, and intimacy. After that, one moved up to the area of esteem needs where accomplishments, prestige and career success would lead to the final stage of self-actualization.

But self-actualization as we said before, is not merely a roadmap to success or feeling powerful. It's about having an inner sense of peace telling you that what you are doing and what you are accomplishing represents YOUR TRUE NORTH. It's leading you to become your true self. It's who you really are.

Yet, so many people identify with the egotistical or even doubting voice in their heads, and many get lost because of this. They spend their lives at the base of the pyramid fulfilling their basic needs, identifying with self-defeating thoughts and beliefs that keep them from climbing higher. But some folks, like avid meditators, use their practice as a way of avoiding this trap.

Current interpretations of the self-actualization pyramid suggest we navigate up and down the pyramid during different times of our lives. We don't always move higher and higher. Certainly, during the pandemic, the whole world moved down to the level of our basic needs for safety, food and water.

During their time in India as young men, right out of college, both Dan Goleman and Richard Davidson suspected there was something remarkably different about the monks, gurus and other life-long meditators they met there. But it took decades of study and research, a lot of which was done back in Dr. Davidson's lab at the University of Wisconsin, to confirm this. In their book, ALTERED TRAITS Goleman and Davidson report: "Now we can share confirmation of these profound alterations of being – a transformation that dramatically ups the limits…of human possibility."[5]

A Tibetan Art Form

A few years ago, four Tibetan Monks, were in residence for one week at a Congregational church in my hometown. They spent that week not only happily interacting with everyone who came to visit, they also spent it creating a large-scale sand painting. Sand paintings are intricate, colorful, beautifully designed artistic compositions that the monks create to shed light on two of the most important concepts of mindfulness: Impermanence and non-attachment.

I visited the church on the fifth day as they were getting near to finishing their work. Just spending time with them was delightful. The sand-painting they were working on was colorful and exquisitely detailed.

At the end of the week, when the Monks were done, they did (and always do) something most Westerners can't even BEGIN to comprehend. They pour the sand painting into a trash bin. We in the West, who save everything we make and or cherish, to the point where many of us become hoarders, find this demonstration of impermanence and non-attachment a bit unnerving. These monks are truly wired differently from the way we are.

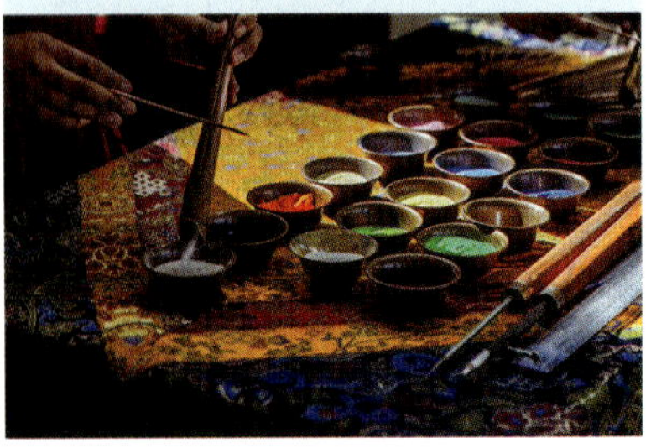

Dr. Paul Ekman, former professor at the University of California at Berkeley, and an advisor to the Disney/Pixar movie about emotions titled, INSIDE OUT, has spent a lifetime studying facial expressions and how our surface expressions reveal our true feelings and emotions. Dr. Ekman's research shows that you can read emotions on a person's face in a fraction of a second and how we often do this subconsciously, without realizing that we're doing it. He has also spent a lot of time studying long-term meditators.

Dr. Ekman says he knows immediately when he meets a long-term meditator. "Their demeanor is different; they are more relaxed. They are unflappable." One of those meditators who Ekman studied was Matthieu Ricard, who we talked about earlier. In a unique experiment, Ekman paired Dr. Ricard in a debate forum with a professor at The University of California at Berkeley who Ekman described as "the second most disagreeable professor" on the UC Berkley campus. (*The most disagreeable professor wouldn't agree to the terms of the debate.*)

This disagreeable professor (who Ekman didn't name) just couldn't ruffle the feathers of Ricard and finally ended up agreeing with Ricard on most of the points of the debate. "I just couldn't argue with this guy, he was too nice," the professor later told Ekman. Next up, Dr. Ekman went to India to spend several days studying the Dalai Lama, who, like all Tibetan Monks, has spent a lifetime meditating. "He is the most authentic person I've ever met," reports Ekman. "There is absolutely no difference between his public persona and his private persona. None whatsoever."[6]

In Malcolm Gladwell's book THE OUTLIERS he writes that "ten thousand hours is the magic number of greatness." Tibetan monks have all spent 10,000 hours plus in meditation. They are without a doubt the elite athletes of the meditation world. When you meet one, you are instantly impressed by how peaceful, serene, and calm they are. They smile easily, laugh easily, make friends easily, but most importantly, and put YOU at ease too, just by being around. I've met maybe a dozen different Tibetan monks in my lifetime, male and female, and they ALL make you feel this way, without exception.

Becoming an elite meditator is certainly not the only path to self-actualization. There's another school of thought that says anyone – who is willing to make a dramatic shift in consciousness – can have access to this higher level of consciousness Maslow named self-actualization. Eckhart Tolle writes about this in his best-selling books THE POWER OF NOW and THE NEW EARTH. "The word enlightenment conjures up the idea of some superhuman accomplishment, and the ego likes to keep it that way, but it is simply your natural state of felt-oneness with Being."[7]

What is a natural state of felt oneness with being? Some people might call it *self-actualization.* Others might call it enlightenment or nirvana or just a state of deep inner peace. It's a place we all want to get to, but for some reason, very few ever do. That's because most of us spend our lives either locked up in our thinking minds, feeling anxious and detached from our surroundings or in a state of perpetual doing, or workaholism, in the desperate hope that "work will set us free." (Ironically these are almost the exact same words posted over the gates of Auschwitz: Work will set *you* free.)

In the next chapter, I think you will discover, what it means to *just* be and feel like you have really *arrived* and know *exactly what it takes to get there.*

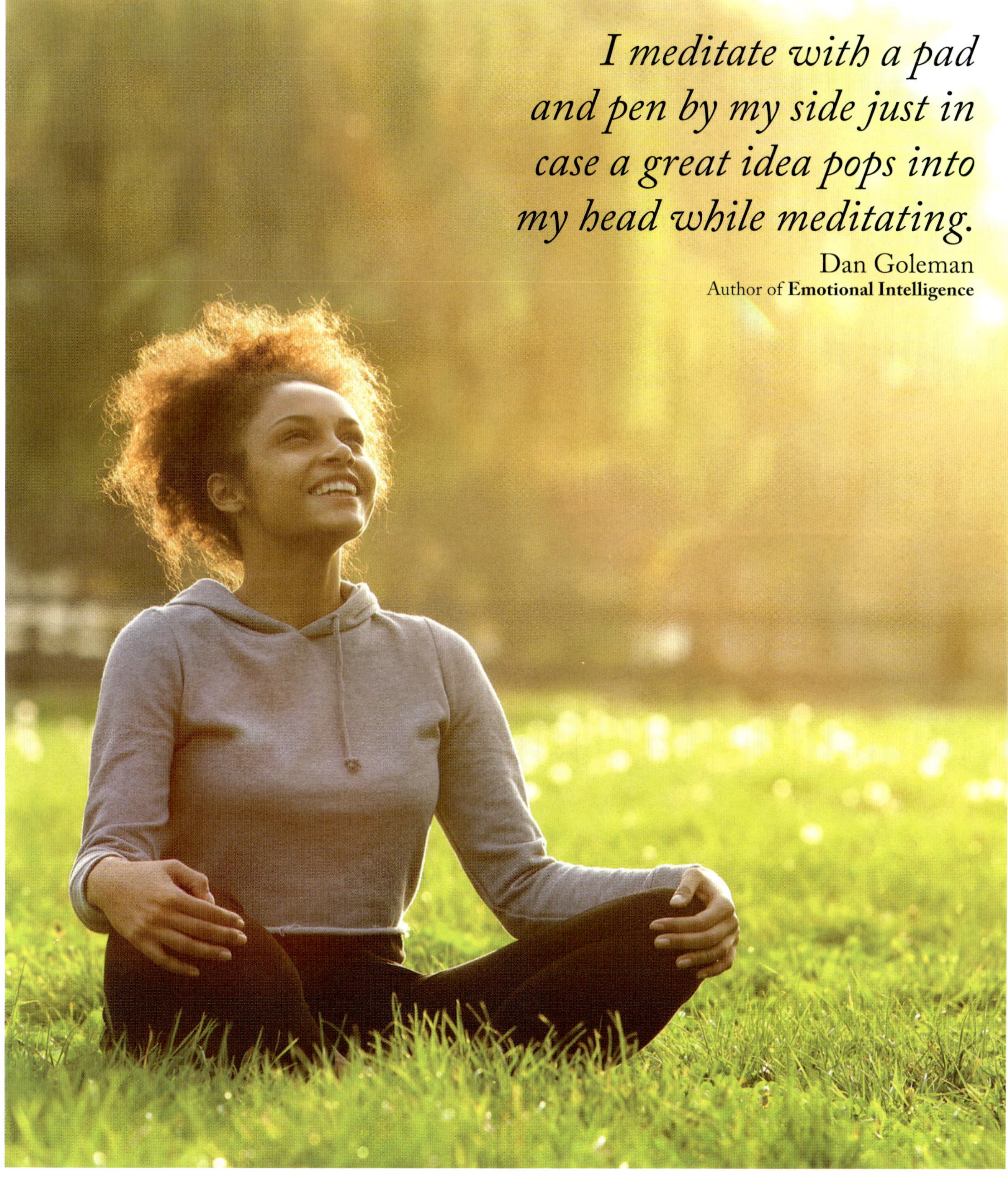
I meditate with a pad and pen by my side just in case a great idea pops into my head while meditating.
Dan Goleman
Author of **Emotional Intelligence**

Chapter 13

On a Mindfulness Retreat

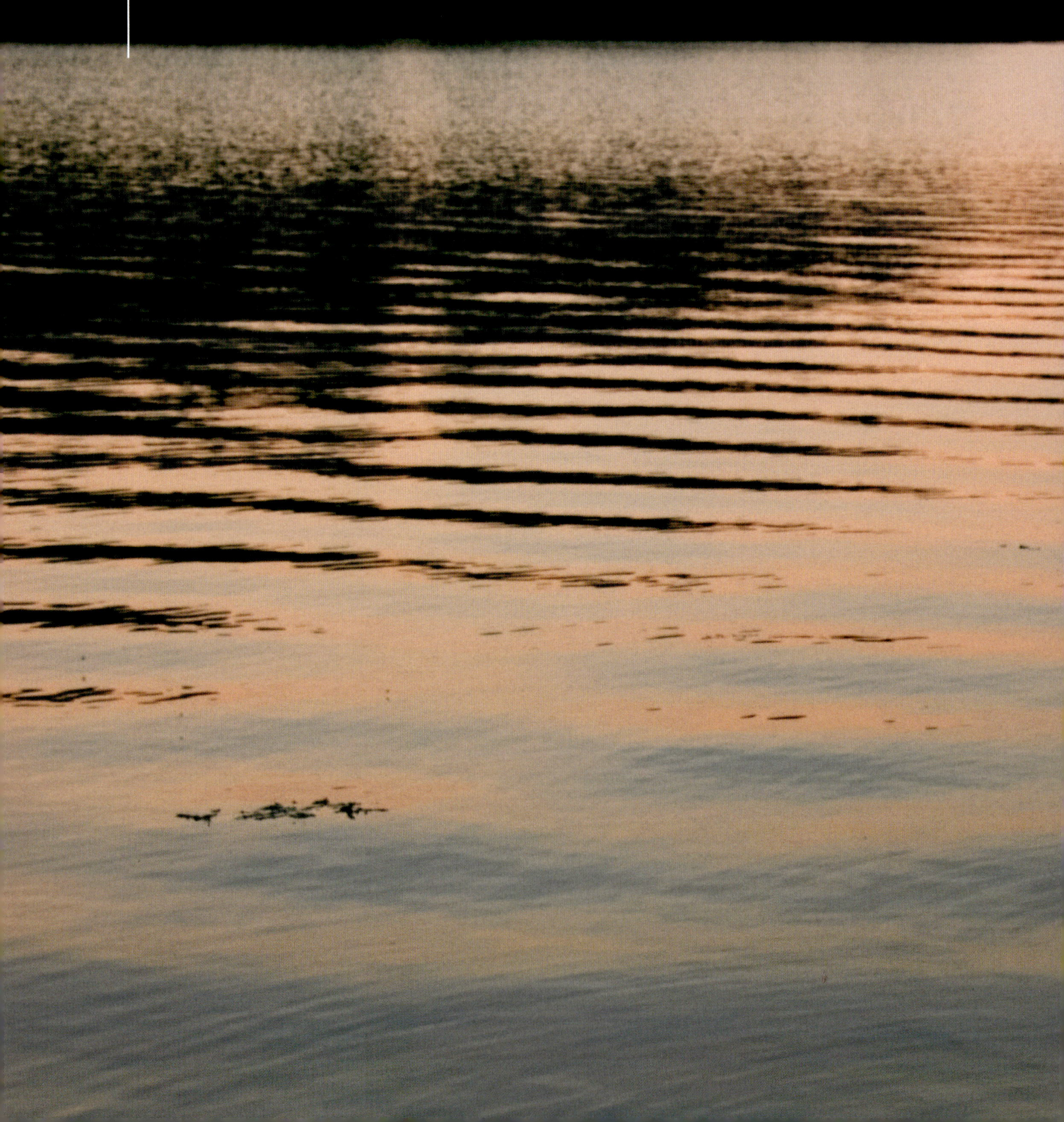

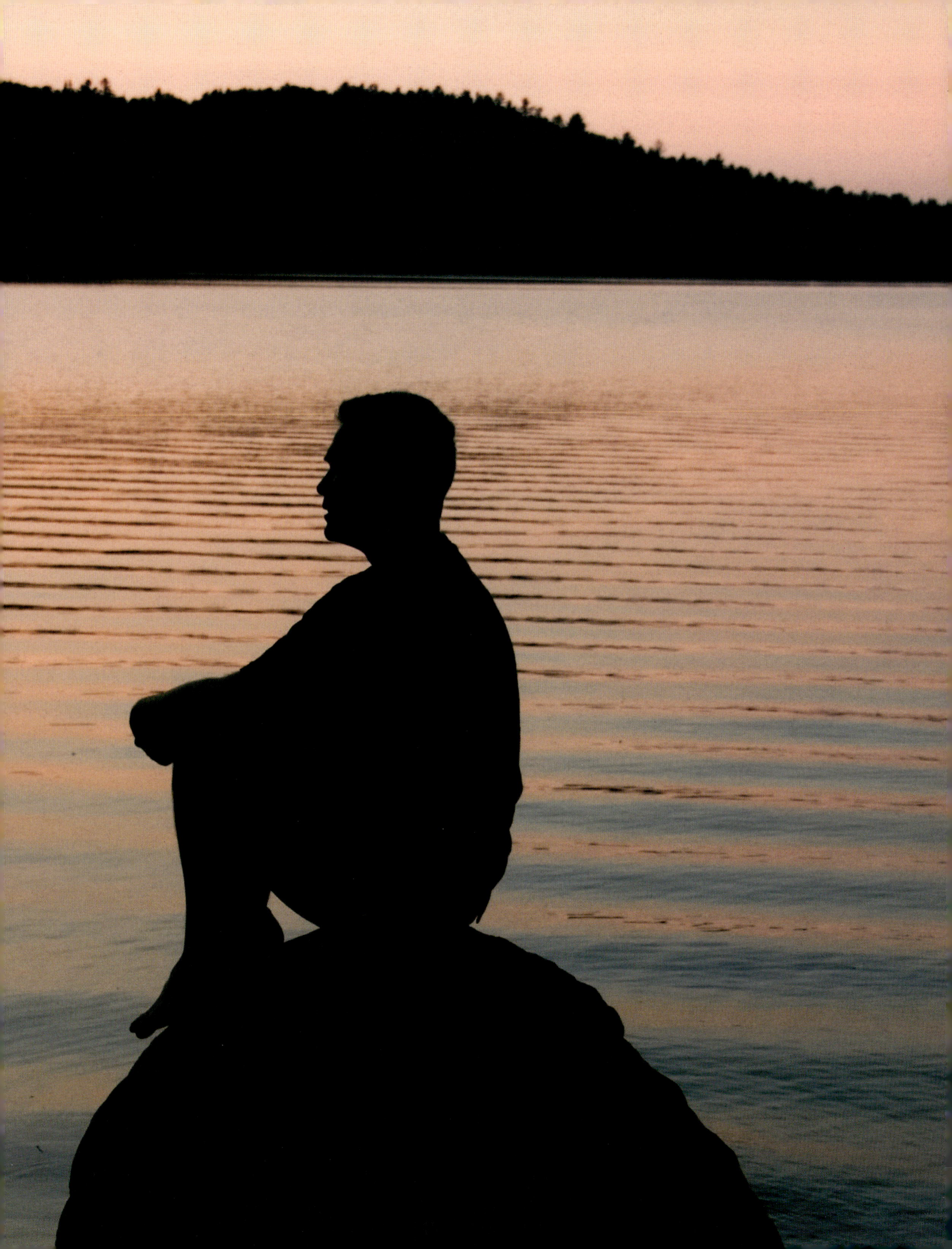

Chapter 13
On a Mindfulness Retreat with Jon Kabat-Zinn

Throughout this book, I've referred to a 6-day mindfulness retreat I went on with Jon Kabat-Zinn. This chapter is based on the diary I kept while on that retreat. I was fairly new to mindfulness at the time, so my observations, are those of a beginning meditator. Some parts of the retreat seemed challenging, other parts seemed strange, and all of it was interesting. Going on a mindfulness retreat is something you might want to consider doing, too. As such, here is a first-hand account, of what it was like for me.

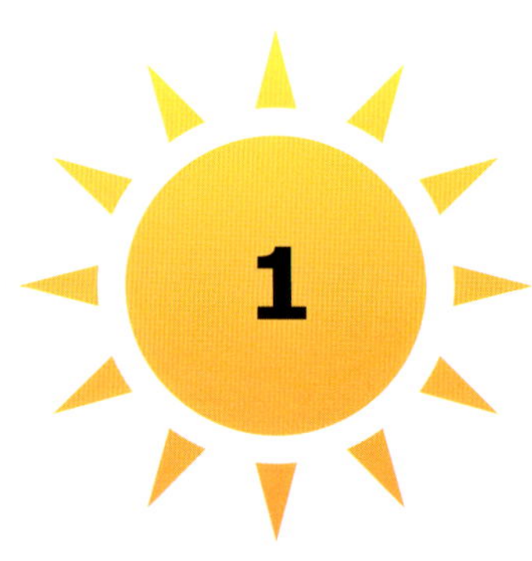

Friday Day 1

As I was walking in the front entrance of Menla Mountain Resort, a Buddhist retreat center in Phoenicia, New York, I was pretty excited to meet Jon Kabat-Zinn. What Michael Jordan or LeBron James is to basketball, Jon Kabat-Zinn is to mindfulness. He has been interviewed by Oprah, Bill Moyers, Anderson Cooper, talked to the Dalai Lama, been on Sixty Minutes, was featured in a cover story in Time Magazine and has been dubbed "Mr. Mindfulness" by the Washington Post. So, when he walked up to me at the registration desk with his short build, his salt and pepper hair and his silver eyebrows jutting up above his wire-rimmed glasses, I recognized him instantly. "Hello," I said, extending my hand, "I'm Jim Porter."

"Hi," he said reaching out to shake mine, "I'm Jon Kabat-Zinn."

The opening session of the retreat took place that night in a Yoga studio, about a half mile down a dirt road. After a vegetarian dinner, the other participants and I walked along the dirt road in the dark, getting to know one another as we tried not to fall into the numerous ruts and ravines we stumbled across along the way. In my group there was a psychiatrist from Nevada, an entrepreneur from San Francisco, and a retired businessman from Ireland.

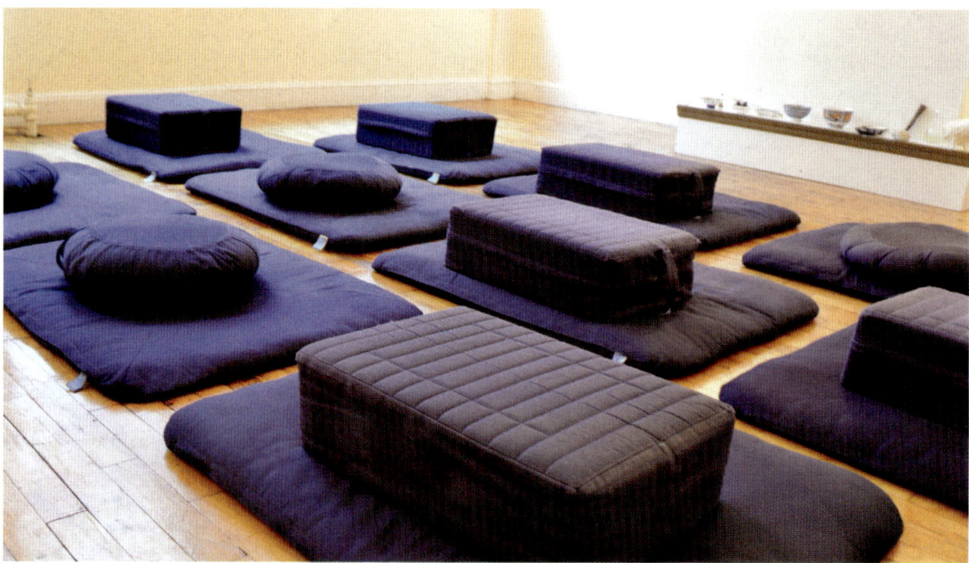

When we had all arrived, or at least thought we had, Jon Kabat-Zinn made a very interesting point. He said: "A lot of you probably haven't even arrived yet. Your bodies are here, but your mind isn't fully here. You may be wondering right now: Did I lock the front door? Did I leave the cat food out? Did I leave the lights on? It may take another 24 hours before your mind has slowed down enough to know that you are really here."[1]

For our first activity, Jon guided us through a visualization where we were all supposed to picture a pebble dropping down a well. When he asked people to comment on the exercise afterwards, one woman volunteered. She said the pebble dropping faster and faster, first through the air, reminded her of her life just before the retreat: So many things to get done before leaving. Hitting the water with a splash represented her arrival at the retreat. The slow descent through the water was the retreat itself. And the pebble landing on the bottom - in the crystal-clear still water - was where she hoped to be by the end of the retreat.

It was such a vivid metaphor for what we were ALL feeling at that moment that everyone's jaw just dropped, in a kind of collective sigh. A middle-aged man sitting in the corner of the room started slowly clapping his hands and the others joined in spontaneously.

Jon Kabat-Zinn interrupted the applause as quickly as it started and announced: "It isn't fair to clap for some people and not for others," he explained, "So I'd prefer it if we didn't applaud at all."

The person who had initiated the applause shot back: "That feels like a put-down." Jon Kabat-Zinn assured him that it wasn't.

Saturday Day 2

The next morning, we assembled in the Yoga Studio, a quarter mile down the dirt road, at 9AM sharp. It was a comfortable space, like a dance studio, about a third the size of a standard gymnasium with a polished wooden floor and windows that looked out on the sloping brown hills that engulfed us on four sides. Inside, there was a circle of 37 blue metal folding chairs and in front of each chair was a matching set of meditation cushions. Thus, each person could choose to sit up in a chair or down on the cushion, also known as a Zafu.

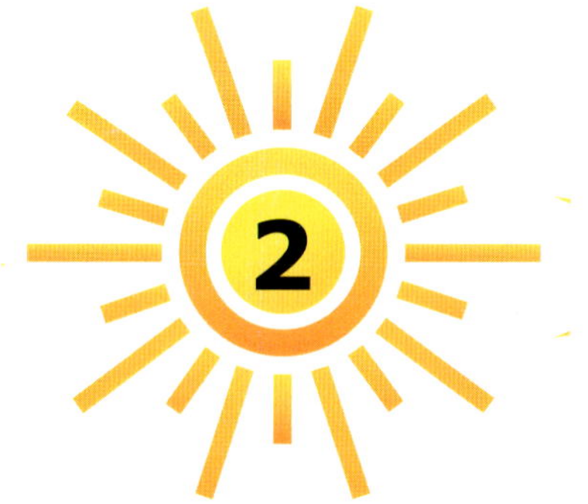

"Welcome," Jon Kabat-Zinn said, sounding truly grateful for our presence in the room. "Just you being here, doing what it takes to get your bodies here in this room is a radical act of kindness, sanity and love."

"Mindfulness is defined as being in the present moment with acceptance," he explained. The goal of mindfulness meditation is simply to be more present with whatever is going on inside you and around you. During the retreat we learned how to do this by focusing our awareness on body sensations, on thinking in a detached way, on environmental sounds, and even through a more mindful practice of yoga. But most of all, we focused on our breathing.

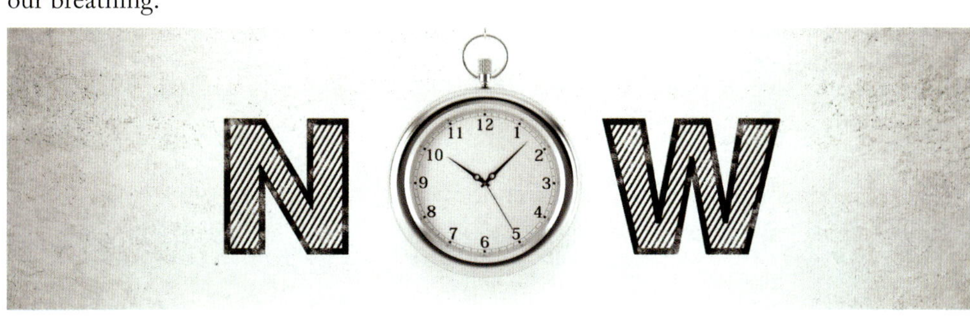

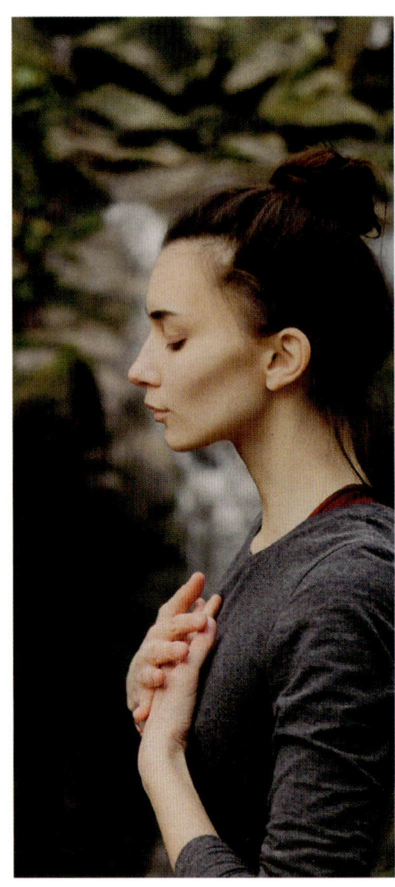

"Bring the breath to center stage, and leave everything else in the wings," Jon Kabat-Zinn said. "If your mind wanders a thousand times away from the breath - and it will - your job is to bring it back a thousand times. And try to throw out the idea of 'Oh, now I'm meditating, or I'm meditating well, or I'm meditating badly.'"

"And don't be too attached to the outcome. Any good scientist knows that attachment to the outcome can ruin an experiment. It can color your results." He didn't seem to want us to go looking for any particular result. It was a bit like a Zen Koan, the short Japanese poems which on the surface don't seem to make any sense: We were to strive without striving, aspire without aspiring and be goal-oriented without caring whether we actually achieved the goal.

After lunch we did our first walking meditation. We were supposed to walk along in super-slow motion trying to concentrate on the rise and fall of each foot along its path from one footfall to the next. Basically, we all looked a bit like zombies doing this. With that thought floating around in the back of my head, I began walking very slowly for ten paces forward and then I'd turn around and walk ten paces back, over and over.

After dinner Jon talked about the philosophy of mindfulness. "We have to be careful not to impose the grid of everything we already know over everything we don't know," he said now talking about the urge to pass judgment on people and activities. "Every second is new by definition." It's not just about being in the present, it's about what results when, in the present, you completely let go of the past. "When you use your ideas about who someone is as a way to disregard them, you're lost." But when you tune into the moment, you see subtle differences that maybe you didn't see before and as the result, conflicts dissolve, arguments don't seem so important and aversion or hate is transformed into a new-found respect.

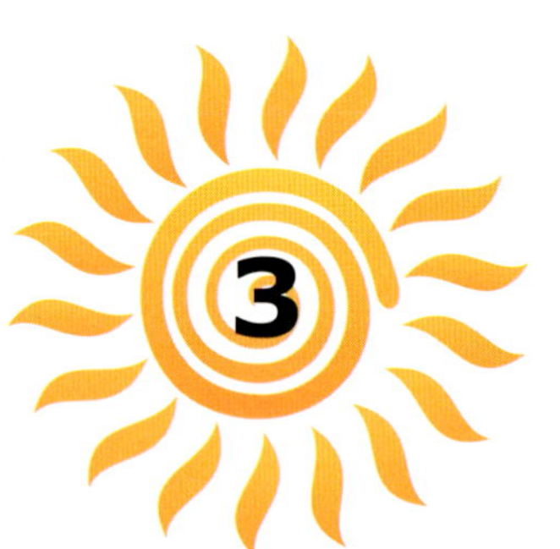

Sunday Day 3

Jon Kabat-Zinn liked to explain, and he could easily take up to a half an hour to answer a single question. That afternoon, someone asked him about how to use mindfulness in the real world.

"Mindfulness increases your personal power," he explained, sounding momentarily like a top-flight sales trainer at a Fortune 500 company. "Your power isn't siphoned off by the need to be right. It isn't sucked up by yesterday's argument and it isn't challenged by tomorrow's fear. Being here right now restores your power, frees you from old arguments and liberates you from fear."

"Being in the moment is about what's happening right now. And every moment is different from the one that just preceded it. So, if something or someone bugged you yesterday, and it's bothering you today, chances are your grasping on to an old story. People love their stories of victimization, poor me, hard luck, difficult spouse, misbehaving children, etc."

"Moment by moment non-judgmental awareness is the key. That way we don't immediately jump into good or bad, black or white, like or dislike. We dwell in the realm (where truth exists) of discernment, of degrees of difference, and subtlety. The mindfulness meditator is less likely to have a story because he or she understands that everyone gets angry, and children misbehave and people let us down, and sometimes things don't go our way, but if it's not happening now, and carries no weight in the present, there's no need to bring it up or even consider it."

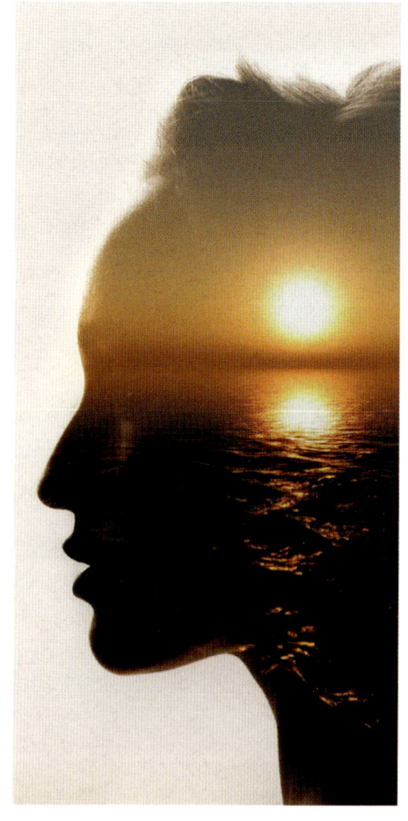

After meditating, Jon always rings his tiny little Tibetan cymbals three times. And at the end of the day he always had some closing words. His words on this third night of the retreat, would lead me, as it turned out, into an experience that was life-changing.

"When you walk out of here tonight, I want you to leave in silence," Jon Kabat-Zinn explained. We will begin our retreat within a retreat - as he liked to call it - tonight and continue it throughout the day tomorrow.

People had been warning me that there was going to be an extended period of silence. And we had practiced this for a meal or two in the first couple of days of the retreat. But I had no idea how severe the restrictions were going to be until Jon Kabat-Zinn laid them out for us that evening. "During this time, I don't want you to talk to anyone, don't look at anyone in the eyes, don't read anything, don't text anyone, don't look at your phones, don’t watch TV and don't use your lap-tops or iPads."

"Can we write on paper?" asked a woman who I think just wanted to hear herself speak one last time.

"No writing. And even when you go to bed, do it mindfully. Be aware of how it feels. Think about being in bed. When you wake up don't jump out of bed. Just lay there for a while and be aware of lying awake in bed. Remind yourself of where you are and what you are doing."

Monday Day 4

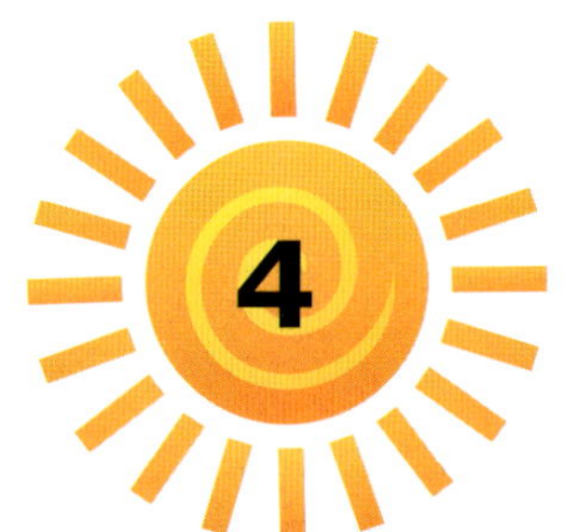

The next morning, I sat directly across from Jon at breakfast. Since we couldn't talk, I found myself strangely fascinated with the contents of his meal tray. There were two small servings of spinach-egg casserole and some strawberries on a white plate and a bowl of oatmeal with a big dollop of yogurt in the middle of the bowl. He ate at a normal tempo - not fast but not slow - and he got up for a second helping afterwards. I later noticed, he always got up for seconds, but he was thin and seemed like he was in good shape. I remember wondering: Can mindfulness boost your metabolism?

When he came back to the table, he turned his chair around, to look out the window, rather than looking at me. Given the fact that we were maintaining "custody of the eyes," (not making eye-contact) I assume he was just being practical.

Even though we had an hour before the next session, I couldn't go read the paper, I couldn't listen to music, I couldn't check my email, I couldn't even phone home. I'd spent a lifetime driven by that voice in the head that says do something, accomplish more, acquire more, don't be lazy. But now, even though that voice wasn't anywhere near silent, it had no reason for being. I could just choose to ignore it, close my eyes, and just BE. So that’s what I decided to try.

The sun came out from behind a cloud and filled my closed eyelids with a kind of orange glow. It reminded me of laying out at the beach in the summer. And it occurred to me that laying out at the beach is one of the few times in life where we allow *being* to take priority over *doing*.

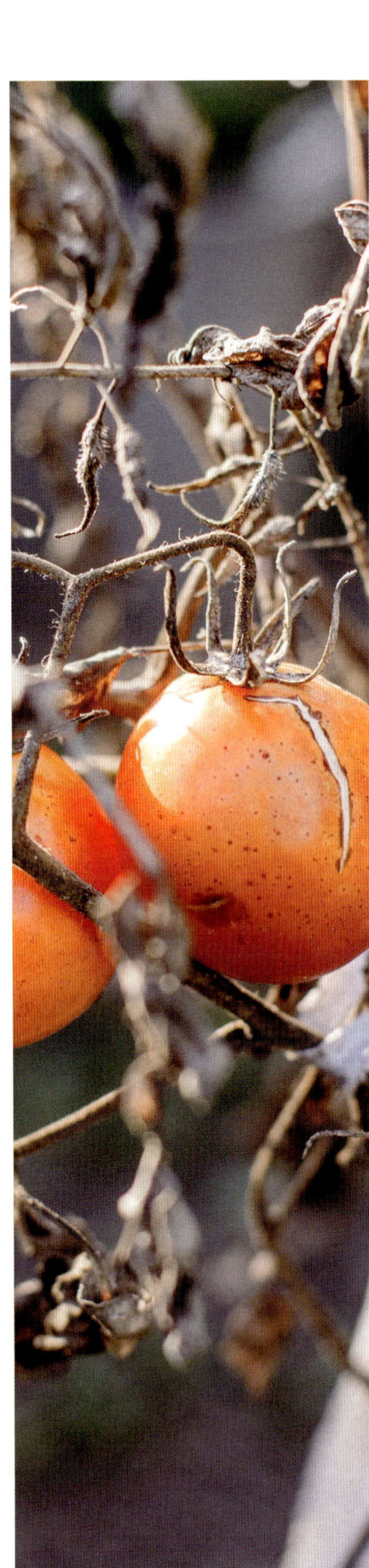

Just then the sun went behind a cloud and the orange glow coming through my eyelids turned into a pale purple. Eventually the purple faded and gradually dissolved into black. I felt like I had been treated to my own all natural, drug-free, mind-made light show. When I finally opened my eyes, it was snowing. Wow!

Since I was in no hurry to DO anything that day, I had plenty of time to think, too. So instead of being caught up in the moment, occasionally thoughts like: Why was I so disconnected from my kids, from my wife and even to some extent from what was going on during this retreat, would ricochet around the seemingly hollow walls of my thick skull. Then the clarifying thought occurred to me, that this was my job as a writer: To be the watcher, the interpreter; to see things through a screen of judgment. But I had gone on this retreat to be *on it*, not to *write about it*. This sense of detachment always left me feeling like I was one step removed from the action: like a person at a dance who never dances.

I walked up to my room, to use the toilet. A sign on the bathroom wall said: "Please use as little TP as possible." In the bathroom, I remembered what Jon Kabat-Zinn had said earlier in the day. "The signature feature of a retreat is there are no breaks. You walk back to your room mindfully and you lay down in bed mindfully and you go to the bathroom mindfully." Was I not being mindful thinking about what he said earlier instead of thinking about what I was doing at that moment? Yes, I thought. But, he also said that as soon as you become aware that your mind has wandered off - you're back in the present. Ah, so I was OK, *for the moment*.

As I walked back down the dirt road to the yoga studio, I noticed an abandoned vegetable garden that, in early November, still had a few tomato vines growing in it. I also noticed two tennis courts that hadn't been played on in a while, and the tarpaulin-covered pool that nobody had been swimming in for months. These reminders of another season made it hard to be in *this season*. All the branches were bare, except for a few tenacious beech trees; each light brown leaf, trembling in the cold wind. Late autumn had a stark beauty all its own, I thought. But it's a beauty that I'd never been able to appreciate before. For some reason, these images had more intensity at this moment and more power. I wondered if the "retreat within a retreat" was beginning to have some sort of positive effect on me: If this is what it meant to have *a felt oneness with being*.

By the afternoon session things began to unravel. My shoulders started to cramp up from all the "sitting" (meditation). Eating meals without being able to smile back at someone seemed like punishment. You couldn't even signal someone to pass the salt and pepper, because that would require making eye-contact.

And then, in the late afternoon session, I noticed a rather loud mouse in the wall. "Isn't anybody else bothered by this darn thing?" I wondered, trying unsuccessfully to block out the sound of the mouse and focus on my breathing. Then there was the coffee pot in the foyer rattling and hissing like an old steam engine. I opened one eye and surreptitiously peered about hoping to find someone looking as irritated as I was. But everyone just kept right on meditating.

Soon it was time to do another Mindfulness walk, and given my state of mind, I wasn't sure I had the patience for it. I decided to walk by myself, away from the rest of the group.

I headed up the road, around the bend, trying to stay mindful. About 15 minutes into my walk, it started to snow, so I cut through the woods – where there was no trail - in order to get back to the yoga studio a little faster. As I walked, I noticed there were apple trees in and amongst other younger trees that had grown up around them. And then right ahead of me, I saw three deer feeding on the apples that had fallen from one of the trees.

I remembered a brochure I'd seen about how the retreat center had been built on the former estate of some rich New York City banker. I guessed that this was once his apple orchard, now buried in the woods where no one could see it, but these deer and me.

As I stopped and stared, I noticed I was feeling more alone and more detached from the whole retreat experience: I missed my family, I missed my friends, I missed talking to people, and I missed looking at people in the eyes.

Then, the flurries changed to a much harder mix of snow and freezing rain. It was coming down hard now in tiny pellets on the earth below. All I could hear was the sound of the icy snow hitting the dry leaves.

As I focused on this surprisingly loud sound, something strange happened. A sense of peace and unity filled me up like I was an empty pitcher being held under a gushing spigot. All my typical doubting, detached thoughts seemed to disappear. *For a moment, I was the sound of icy snow hitting the leaves.*

In an instant, I thought about these woods and its history, and I wondered how many people had stood in this exact spot before me: I was just as much the owner of this spot as the Menla Mountain House, or the rich New York City banker, or the Native Americans who preceded us all. These random images were flowing over me in a unified way that I didn't make any attempt to label. It was an indescribable feeling that had magically emerged out of a bucket load of pain.

Months before, I had read in Eckhart Tolle's book, THE POWER OF NOW, about fleeting moments of pure bliss, called Satori, that could occur spontaneously, out of the blue. Tolle defined it as a moment of enlightenment where you get a temporary glimpse of what it might feel like to BE enlightened. The moment ended as quickly as it began but when it was over, I KNEW I had experienced something special: I had felt completely connected to and was ONE with the world around me and then, as fast as it came, it was gone.

By the time I returned to the studio, everyone was inside including Jon Kabat-Zinn who was beginning to speak about non-attachment. The coffee maker was gurgling away, and the mouse was busy doing his acrobatics in the wall, but suddenly that didn't seem to matter to me anymore.

Tuesday Day 5
The next morning after breakfast, we broke the silence and the floor was wide open for questions. "Is there a bag of tricks you can give us to take back home?" a woman from Denmark asked, who I had accidentally made eye-contact with during the silence.

"What does the sign say at a Railroad Crossing?' Jon Kabat-Zinn asked back.

"I don't know, I'm from Denmark," and everyone in the room laughed except Jon.

"It says: stop, look, listen," Jon Kabat-Zinn replied, always ready for the next moment.

The Guest House

Around the fourth day of the retreat, Jon Kabat-Zinn started reading poetry to us. This one, written in the 13th century by a Sufi poet named Rumi, seems to be everyone's favorite mindfulness poem, including mine:

This being human is a guest house.
Every morning a new arrival.
A joy, a depression, a meanness,
some momentary awareness comes
As an unexpected visitor.

Welcome and entertain them all!
Even if they're a crowd of sorrows,
who violently sweep your house
empty of its furniture,
still treat each guest honorably.
He may be clearing you out
for some new delight.

The dark thought, the shame, the malice,
meet them at the door laughing,
and invite them in.

Be grateful for whoever comes,
because each has been sent
as a guide from beyond.

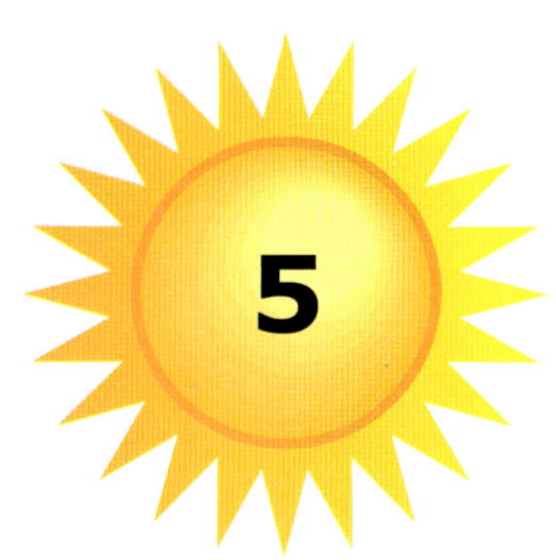

"Right in the middle of losing your mind there are lots of things you can do," he continued, now apparently on a roll. "You can: 1. Just flip out. 2. Get your "butt" and put it on a cushion," he said, now sprinkling in a curse word or two for the first time during the retreat. "Do something to change the place you're in. Take a break. Remind yourself, life goes on, I'm still alive. 3. Listen deeply. 4. Stop, really stop. Even if you think you don't have time to - that's probably just mind-created anyway - remember the law of impermanence. Everything changes. Your anger, your crazy mood, your strong emotions will all go away."

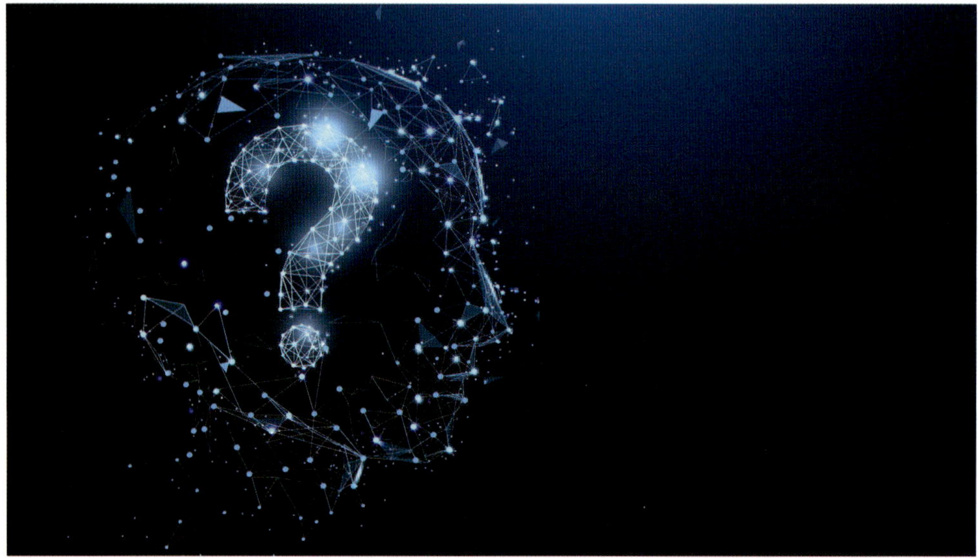

"Do I need to meditate every day for 45 minutes?" asked a young guy from New Jersey in a flannel shirt.

"Try to meditate for 10 minutes a day and see how much you get back. This practice is entirely empirical. It's got to work for you, or it doesn't work at all. When we sit, this is where we hone our skills. We get better at understanding our thoughts and being aware of our emotions. How they're linked and how we can separate who we are from them."

"How much time do you spend meditating?" I asked him, wondering if he'd take issue with this question.

"I don't want to reify my practice," he said back-peddling a bit, "then you'll all try to imitate me rather than figure out what's best for you. But what I am willing to say is: for forty years I got up at 5AM every morning and did a combination of yoga and meditation for two hours every day."

A former Madison Avenue advertising executive shouted out. "I just got three pieces of bad news, and to be honest, I'm not sure how I'm supposed to handle it?" He clearly sounded agitated. "What did I learn over the last 36 hours of silence that I'm supposed to apply to that bad news?"

Whenever there was a tough question, or one that had some emotion attached to it, Jon would take a deep breath in, breath out, think for a minute and just let the words of the questioner hang in the air. And when he was good and ready, he would answer. "The whole world is collaborating in your education - your curriculum. It might help to take the bad news and put the welcome mat out for it. Your mind is already making up stories and maybe they're not accurate."

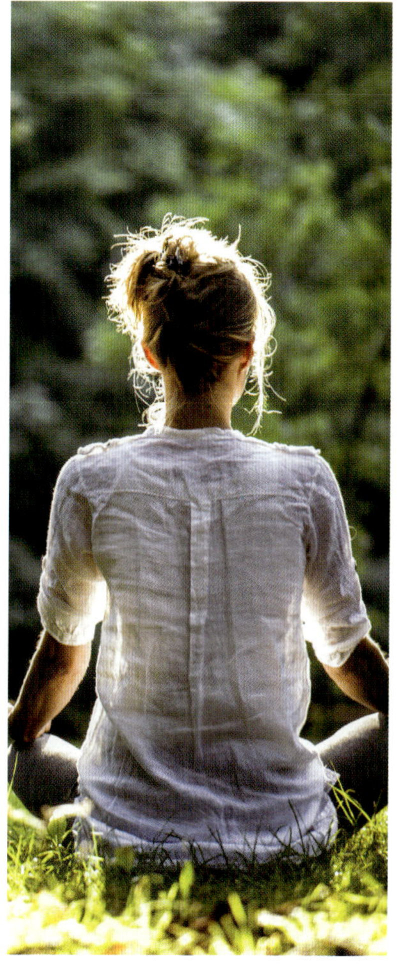

At the end of that afternoon session and what was now getting to be the waning hours of our retreat, we did the Mountain Meditation. I had been told that this was Jon's signature meditation exercise for an MBSR retreat. It was a lesson about the concept of impermanence, that everything changes all the time. But it was also a lesson about being resilient in the face of that impermanence. Now that most of us were able to sit in the full or half lotus position, with our legs folded, knees on the floor, the observation that we resembled mountains seemed truly plausible.

"Imagine your arms are like the sloping sides of the mountain and your head is like the high peak. The whole body is majestic and magnificent. We sit in stillness like mountains. The seasons change, the weather changes, people come and go, but the mountain remains unchanged. Storms swirl around the mountain, but the mountain is always grounded, always rooted in the earth, always still. The mountain shows us that we can be stable and balanced in the face of the emotional storms in our own minds and bodies."

At the end of the meditation I felt like I had finally gotten it. Mindfulness was about a lot of things - not just about being in the moment. It was about acceptance of what is, it was about not passing judgment, not clinging to old ideas and it was about not resisting the inevitable flow of change. When we are inside our thinking brain - as most of us are 24/7 - our thoughts and emotions rule the day.

But below that thinking brain was our mountain, our awareness, our knowing that everything we in the West hold so dear: our cars, our jobs, our stainless-steel kitchen appliances, were all like the weather and the changing seasons on top of that mountain. It was all as ephemeral as falling leaves. But the mountain is unchanging, unalterable, and never-ending.

Wednesday Day 6
After breakfast, Jon was in no hurry to move into whatever activity would be the last activity of the retreat. Finally, he rang his little Tibetan cymbals and asked: "How many people in the room will have a person or persons waiting for them when they get home?" Most of the hands went up. "Imagine this person and what they are doing right now. Remember people at home and at work may not have missed you but instead may be resenting all the work they had to do while you were gone."

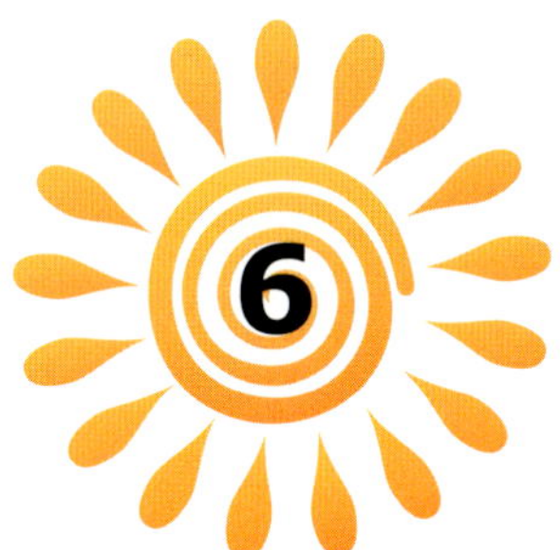

"And when they ask you what you did on this retreat it may be best to say as little as possible. They probably don't want to hear that you meditated, laid around, ate gourmet meals, did yoga for six days and still managed to suffer. They just won't get it. So just don't tell them anything. Or if they really press, just tell them we meditated a lot."

It was about 10:30 and the retreat was going to end in less than an hour, whether we wanted it to or not. And there was this palpable sense in the room that everyone was hoping that it wouldn't end. Jon opened the floor to anyone who wanted to make a closing statement.

An older woman, who was wearing a green wool coat like my Grandmother used to wear, said she'd realized something very profound. In a shaky voice she said: "When I arrived

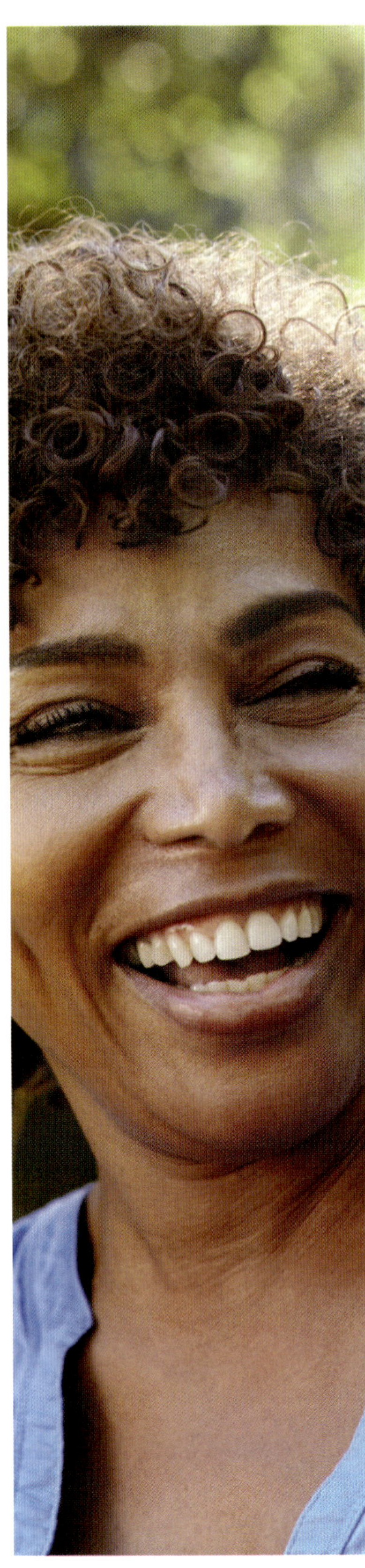

on Friday, Jon, I'd come here for you. You were my teacher. But yesterday I realized I was not here for you. I was here for me."

And without hesitating Jon responded: "It's about time you realized that."

A frail looking older gentleman (I guessed to be in his late seventies or early eighties) said he wanted to recite a poem he'd memorized from one of Jon's books:

"The birds have vanished..." he began, and then stopped, choking on his own words.

He started again, this time, his voice barely above a whisper, almost as if he were talking from his deathbed.

"The birds have vanished into the sky
and now the last cloud drains away.
We sit together the mountains and me.
Until only the mountains remain."

Some people looked sad, some people were sniffling, and others were just sobbing outright. I had to admit, even formerly jaded old me, was holding back tears. At that point a bright-faced woman from Miami, who seemed like the happiest person I'd ever met, just started singing out loud: *There's a smile on my face. For the whole human race. And it's almost like being in love.*

She sang the whole song from start to finish in a perfect soprano voice and in perfect tune. And when she was done the whole room broke out in spontaneous applause for what was only the second time during the entire retreat.

Epilogue

It's been many years since I went on that retreat and now, with the benefit of hindsight, I can honestly say: it was a valuable investment with a very specific benefit. Before the retreat, I was enamored with mindfulness, but I didn't have a meditation practice in place. After the retreat I started meditating just about every day.

And that has really changed me. We talked in an earlier chapter about state changes (what you feel while meditating) vs. trait changes (what you feel as the RESULT of meditating). And it's those trait changes that add up, little by little, over time. As a person who meditates now, usually for about a half an hour every day, I can feel the change inside me. I'm happier. I'm less moody. Even my children can see it. My son calls me "the Zen master." And now my wife has started calling me "Buddha Jim." What more proof do you need that mindfulness really works than that?

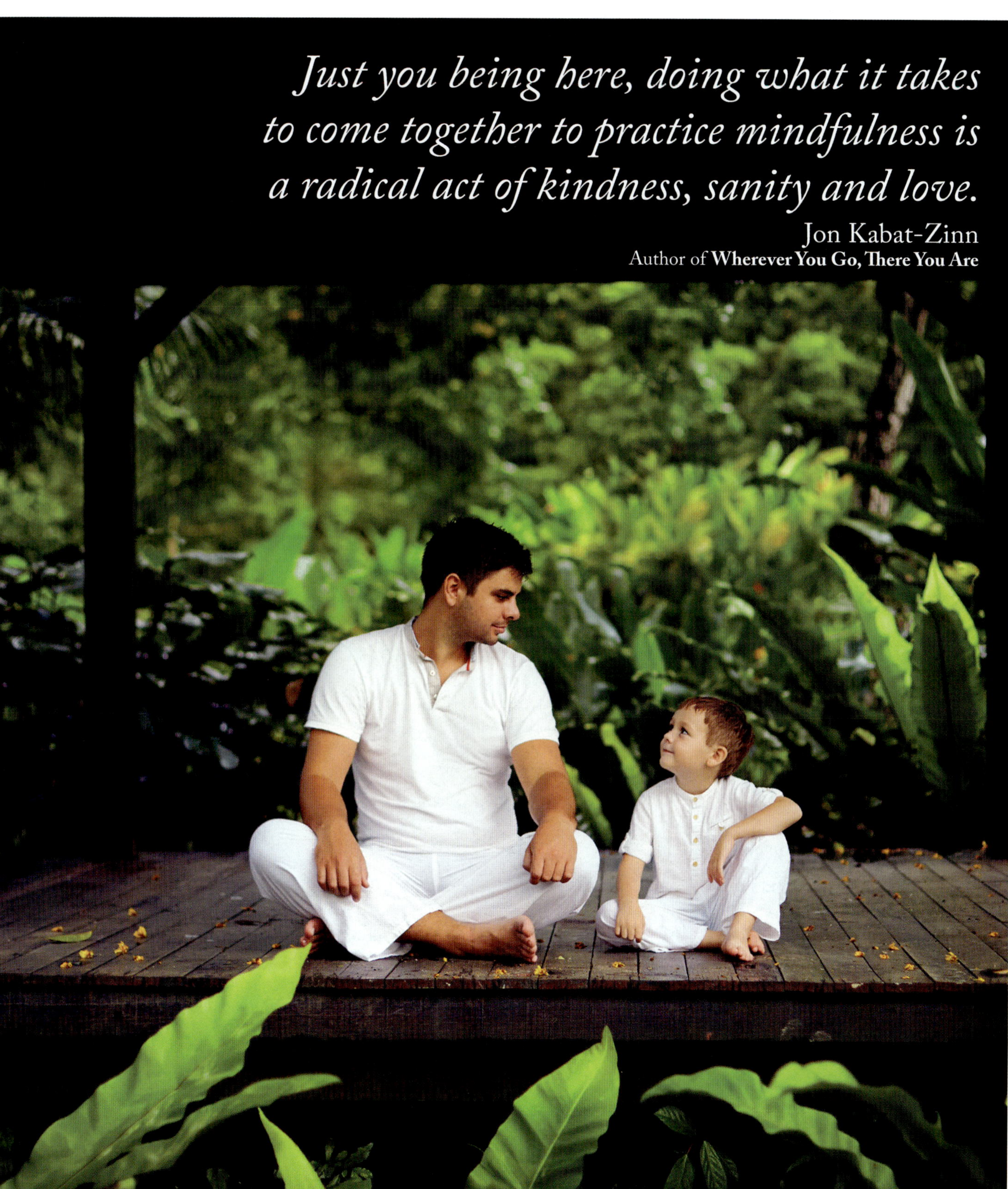
Just you being here, doing what it takes to come together to practice mindfulness is a radical act of kindness, sanity and love.
Jon Kabat-Zinn
Author of **Wherever You Go, There You Are**

Chapter 14

Become Aware of Your Awareness

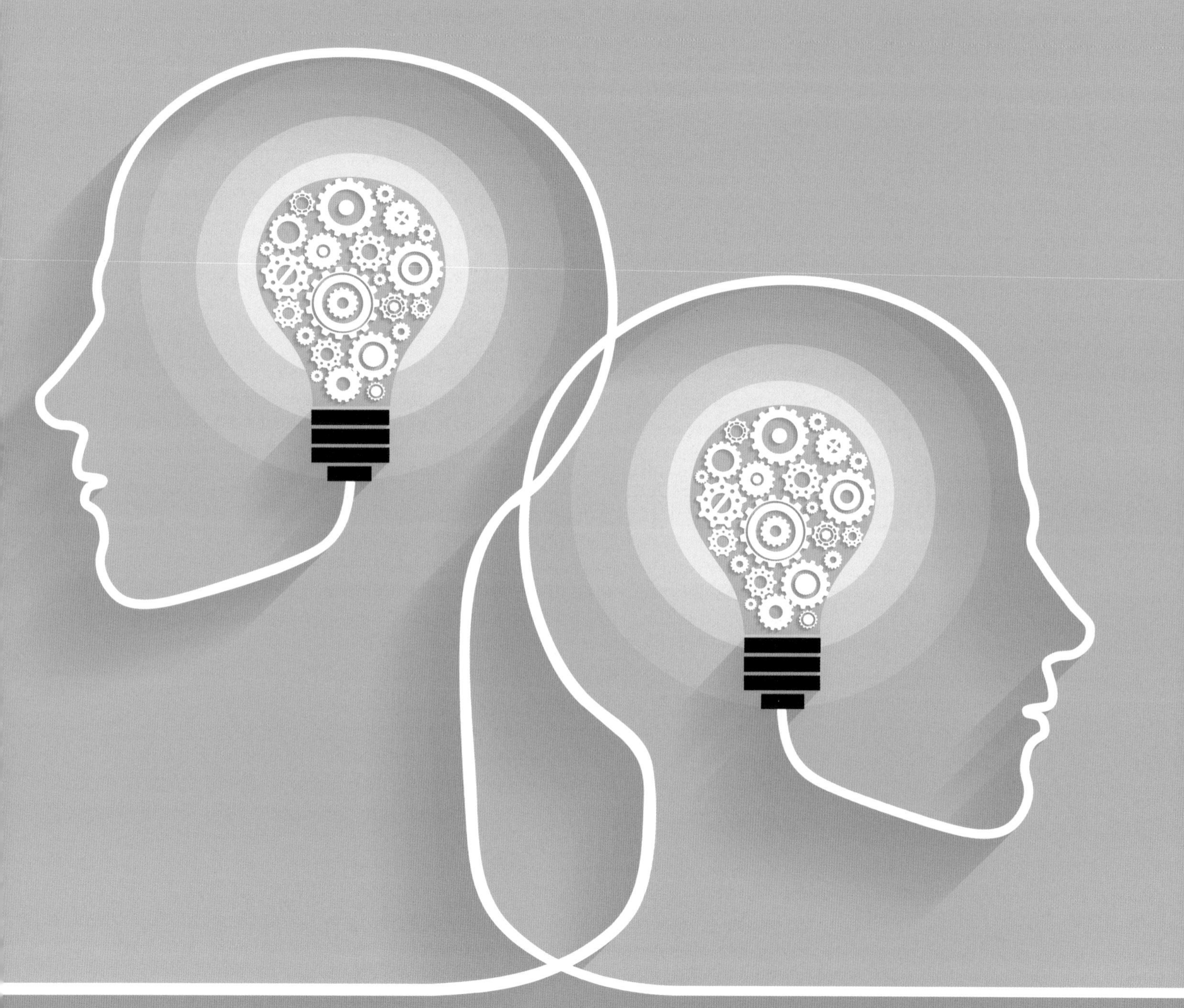

Chapter 14
Become Aware of Your Awareness

Even though I wrote the previous chapter years ago, based on notes I took during the retreat, I was surprised to see there is not one single mention in this account of the line: *Awareness doesn't get angry, awareness doesn't get anxious, awareness doesn't get depressed.* Yet, as I'm sure you remember, in Chapter 1, I concluded that this was the most important takeaway from the entire retreat. Why didn't I include it here in this diary, originally written right after the retreat concluded?

In looking back, I think the reason I didn't include it was that I wasn't sure if I had heard it right, or if he had said it at all. At first, it didn't even make any sense to me. Then, while recently reading "Altered Traits" by Dan Goleman and Richard Davidson, I came across what must have been the ACTUAL quote, written by an author named Sam Harris. As it turns out, the quote is slightly different: "That which is aware of sadness, is not sad. That which is aware of fear, is not fearful."

Maybe Jon Kabat Zinn said it the way I remembered it, or more likely, he was quoting Sam Harris exactly at the time and I heard it differently. So I think I didn't include the quote in my original account of the retreat, because I hadn't specifically written it down in my notes, and I was still a bit mystified by it after the retreat was over.

Either way, what we are talking about here is referred to in mindfulness as *meta-awareness.* Earlier in the book I mentioned psychologist and author Albert Ellis who wrote: "Mankind is the only animal that can think about his thinking." Thinking about your thinking is called *meta-cognition.* When you are aware of your awareness that's *meta-awareness.* And this is truly what mindfulness is all about: meta-awareness. After you put down this book, I want you to always remember: *To be aware of your awareness.*

Everything you do can be done with this extra measure of awareness: While folding the laundry, while putting away the dishes, while driving to work, while at work, while talking to someone, and certainly while meditating. When you do your life in this way, the neural pathways in your brain for controlling negative thoughts and emotions will become stronger and stronger. The more you practice both informal and formal mindfulness, the more benefits you will accrue from it like improved focus, less stress, and better health. In other words, the more you practice *meta-awareness* both while sitting (meditating) and throughout your day, the better you will get at it.

There's an age-old Zen expression that applies here: *Before enlightenment you chop wood and carry water. After enlightenment you chop wood and carry water.* If the ultimate goal of mindfulness meditation is enlightenment and nothing changes afterwards, what's the point of it? Well, after enlightenment your chores no longer feel like chores. Everything you do is a meditation because you do it with meta-awareness.

Remember what I said about automaticity back in chapter 1? Automaticity is our ability to do things on autopilot and what ultimately leads us to doing things mindlessly. In other words, over time we learn to ride a bike or drive a car or operate a computer without even thinking about it. So it may come as a surprise to learn that automaticity can be a good thing as it applies to learning how to meditate.

When is it OK or GOOD to leave the present moment?

Typically, when we leave the present moment, we do so because our mind wanders. As a result, the task we are working on, the friends we are talking to, or the operation we are performing (like driving a car) doesn't get our full attention. This form of mindlessness leads to accidents, mistakes, hurt feelings and the misery of constantly worrying about the future or not letting go of the past.

But YES, there are times when we NEED to leave the present moment. Maybe you are planning a party, or a wedding and you need to consider what might happen if your liberal Uncle Andrew sits at the same table as your conservative cousin Edgar. But this isn't mind-wandering. You are purposefully using your mind like a tool, to help you consider what might or might not happen in the future and then making conscious decisions based on what you predict.

I have a friend who is an avid meditator. He is allergic to Novocain and prefers not to take any form of pain medication when he goes to the dentist. He tells me when he gets a cavity filled, he just takes his mind somewhere else, and says the pain is quite manageable.

When you first learn something, the area of the brain that pilots the new activity is the prefrontal cortex (PFC). Learning something new requires a lot of effort and thinking power. Once you get the hang of it, these skills gradually become automatic. When that happens, control of the activity moves from the PFC down to the brain stem, or the basal ganglia which, if you get good enough, allows you to do the new activity without having to think that much about it at all. In other words, *with much less mental effort.*

The same is true of mindfulness meditation. When you first start meditating, it requires a lot of effort. Your prefrontal cortex struggles to keep extraneous thoughts from coming into your mind. But new research – coming out of Richard Davidson's lab – shows that automaticity eventually kicks in as we get better and better at meditating. The more experienced you get, the less effort your meditation will require.[1]

Start a meditation practice today. Even if it's as little as two minutes a day. You can build slowly from there. Don't make the mistake of thinking you are going to start out meditating an hour a day, just because you read this book. Start small.

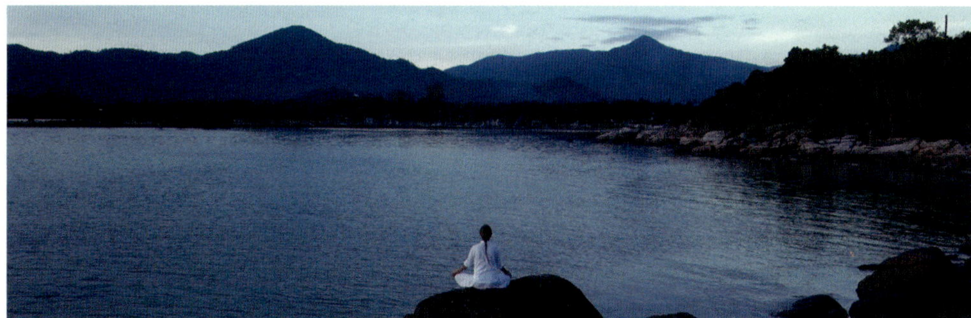

Most people begin their formal mindfulness meditation practice by focusing on their breathing. Notice every inbreath, every outbreath and notice the gap between your outbreath and the next inbreath. Mindfulness meditation can be as simple as that. Really zero in on when your mind wanders. Get to know when you are meditating and when you are not. This was surprisingly helpful for me at first to firmly establish what constitutes mind-wandering. That's why I spent so much time spelling it out in Chapter 2.

Your formal practice of meditation will inform and inspire your informal practice of being out in the world. You'll get better and better at staying in the moment all day long. You can start your informal practice by learning to savor moments in the shower, while eating, while listening, while working on a project that fully engages your attention, and while out in nature. These are all times where it will be just a bit easier to *pay attention on purpose.*

Use your meditation practice to help you fall asleep at night, or to create a boundary between work and home, or to unlock your creative mind. Remember how Dan Goleman likes to meditate with a pad and pen next to him? Solutions to problems and good ideas often pop into my head while meditating. When this happens I quickly write the thought or idea down and go back to meditating.

Remember, mindfulness is as much a philosophy as it is a practice. Terms like acceptance, non-judgment and non-attachment are all reminders of how a different philosophical view, can help us find peace in this world. Understand that ego, attraction, aversion, craving, and putting off happiness until some future date are all obstacles that can get in the way of finding this peace.

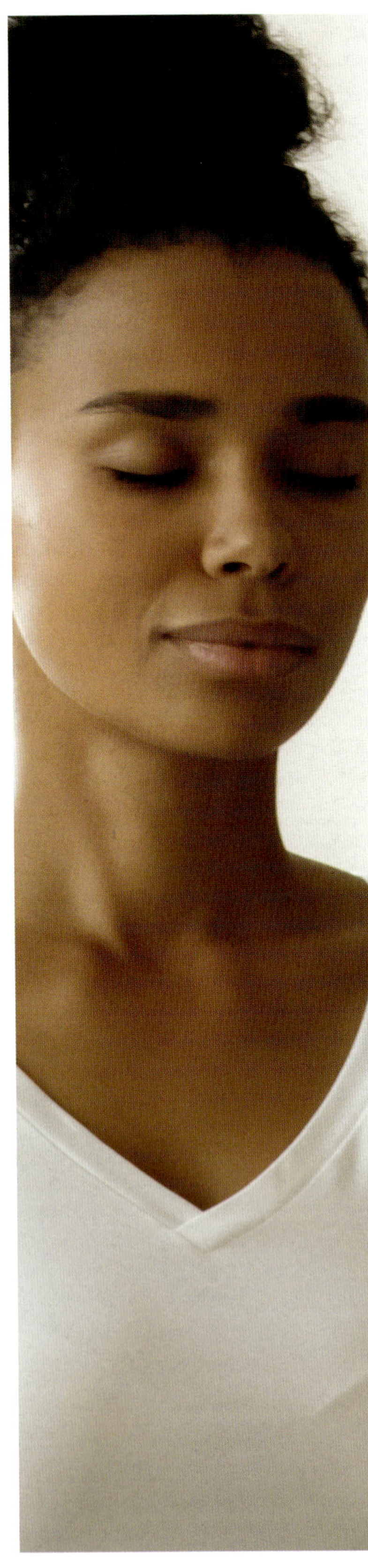

Keep in mind that the many benefits of mindfulness practice from help dealing with pain, lowering stress, boosting your immune system, improving your concentration, to changing the very structure of your brain come from continued practice. The more you practice the more locked in these benefits become. As Dan Goleman likes to say: The larger the dosage, the greater the effect.

That said, many of the benefits of mindfulness – particularly the inner peace it can bring – are all available to you *right now*. They are all locked into this *very* moment – the only moment you can ever experience – which is right here and right now. Allow me to end this book with an old mindfulness cliché, which even if you've heard before, you can't help but see the wisdom in it: Yesterday is history. Tomorrow is a mystery. But this moment is a gift. That's why it's called the *present*.

Ten key points to remember:

1. **Meditation changes the very structure of your brain.** Research out of Harvard, by Dr. Sara Lazar, has shown that your brain starts to change as your meditation practice progresses. Areas of the brain responsible for emotional control get bigger and areas of the brain responsible for emotional outbursts get smaller.[2]

2. **Your mind is going to wander.** When it does, bring it back to whatever it is you are focusing on like your breathing. Remember, this is like doing reps at the gym. You're strengthening the muscle of concentration.

3. **There's no such thing as a bad meditation.** As long as you keep trying to bring your mind back into the present moment, *without judgment*, you are going to get something out of your meditation.

4. **You DO have time to meditate.** Even a minute here or two minutes there will do you some good.

5. **The more you meditate the easier it gets.** Richard Davidson's research proves this.[3]

6. **The present moment is a refuge from both anxiety and anger.** It's when we leave the present moment and worry about the future that we get anxious. And it's when we leave the present moment and review the bad things that have happened in the past that we get upset.

7. **Acceptance is a gateway to the present moment.** If you are upset by something that has already happened, until you let that go, you will be locked out of the joy of living in the present moment.

8. **Acceptance hack.** When you *can't* accept something, *accept that you can't accept it.*

9. **The story of the two arrows:** The first arrow is the real pain. The second arrow is your story around the pain. Learn to control the pain of the second arrow and that may help you control the pain of the first arrow too.

10. **State effects vs. trait effects.** State effects are what you feel while meditating: You might feel happy, relaxed, at one with the world. Trait effects are what happens as the result of meditating: you learn to concentrate better, your startle response diminishes, you gain control over your emotions.

12 Month Meditation Schedule

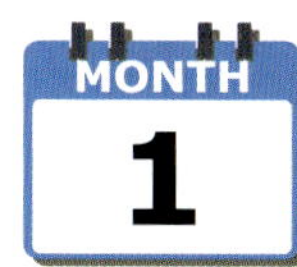

Start by practicing meditation 5 minutes a day when you first wake up. Try each one of the ten meditations from chapter 2 in this first month. Figure out which ones you like the best. Try to notice the difference between when you are doing things mindfully and when you are doing things mindlessly. If you wake up in the middle of the night, try meditating until you feel sleepy.

Favorite meditation style

Second favorite meditation style

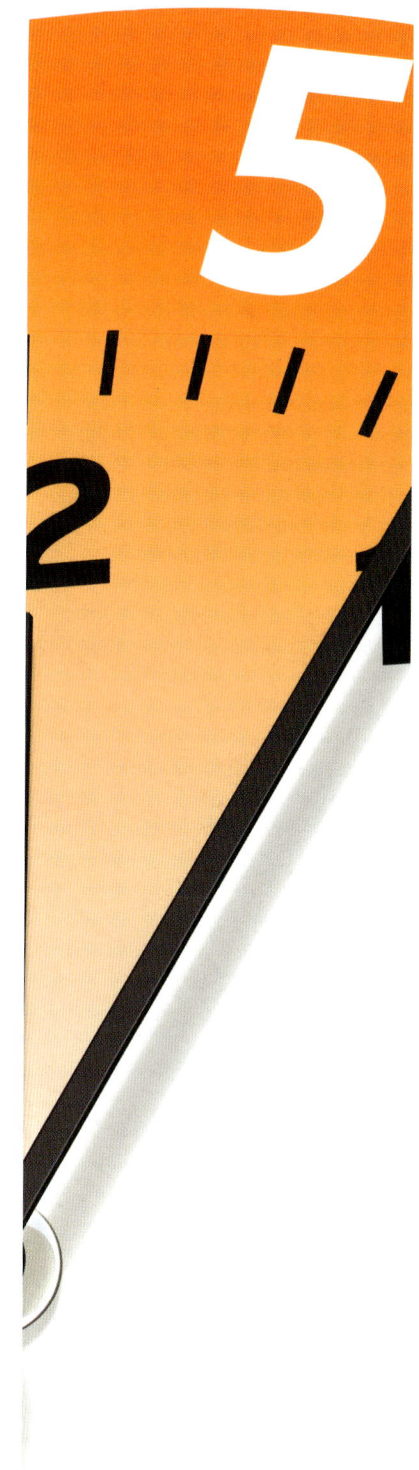

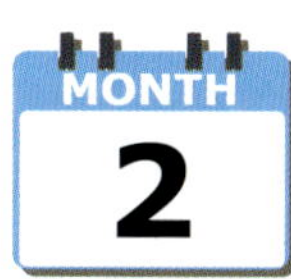

Add in one more 5-minute mindfulness meditation during lunch, or when you come home from work or before you go to bed. Do the meditation you like the best first thing in the morning. Continue trying out the other styles of meditation mentioned in Chapter 2 during your second meditation period. In addition, find 5 activities at home or work, where *paying attention on purpose* comes more easily. If you can, do more and more of these mindful activities this month.

Activities that easily hold my attention:

1.

2.

3.

4.

5.

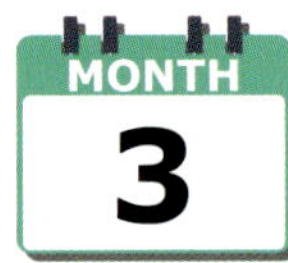

Try adding a 20 to 30-minute meditation once a week, to your two 5-minute sessions. Check off 3 things from chapter 5 that you can do at work to integrate mindfulness into your daily routine and see if you can do at least one of them every day at work this month.

1.

2.

3.

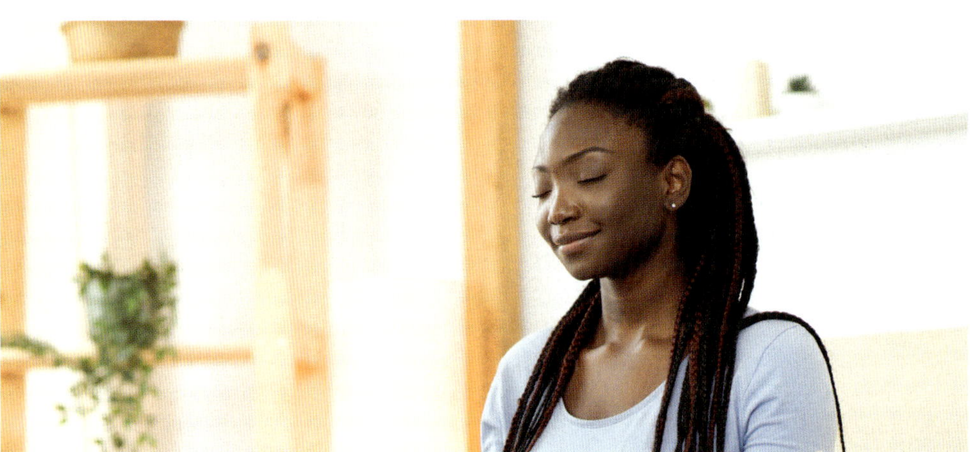

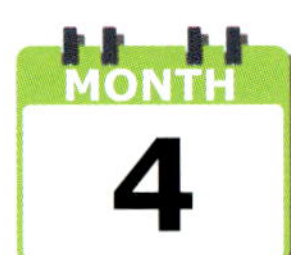

Try squeezing a third 5-minute session into your day or add an additional 5 minutes to your morning meditation. Notice the difference between when you're meditating and when you're not, which I wrote about in Chapter 2. Go back to that chapter and find 3 additional tips that will help you with your meditation this month.

1.

2.

3.

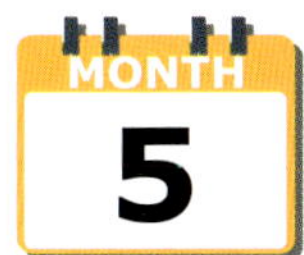

Add in one more 20 to 30-minute meditation per week, for a total of two long meditations per week. Try also adding in a Loving Kindness Meditation to your routine for one week this month. (See sidebar in Chapter 2) The research suggests this meditation method yields fast results. Alternately, make a list below of five things you have to be grateful for and repeat them silently to yourself before going to sleep at night.

1.

2.

3.

4.

5.

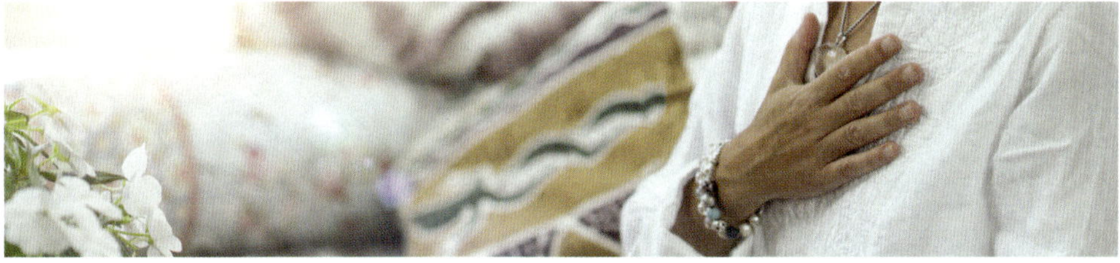

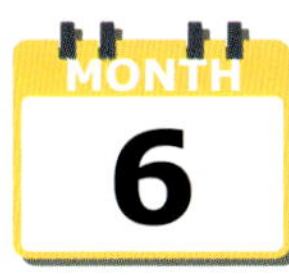

You are now meditating 15 minutes a day. And adding in two longer meditations a week of 15-20 minutes each. Reread chapter 4 on the ten ways to use mindfulness philosophy in your daily life. Choose three things from that chapter that you think would help you be more mindful this month.

1.

2.

3.

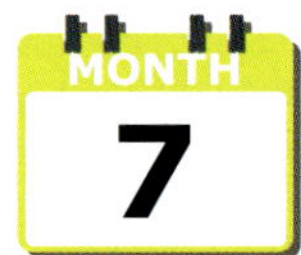

You've now been meditating for 6 months. Congratulations! Keep up with your 15 minutes a day of practice (with the two longer 20 to 30-minute sessions per week) and don't change a thing. Once a week this month think of three examples of situations you handled more gracefully than you might have handled them before you started meditating.

Month 7 Week 1

1.
2.
3.

Month 7 Week 2

1.
2.
3.

Month 7 Week 3

1.
2.
3.

Month 7 Week 4

1.
2.
3.

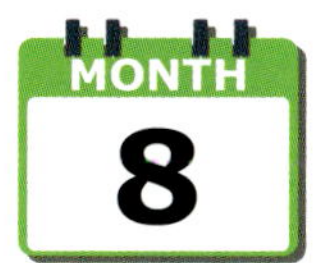

If you think you are ready to add another 5 minutes to either your morning or evening routine, do so. In addition, think of three examples of issues you are having trouble resolving and write them down in the spaces below. Before one of your long meditation sessions, ask yourself: How can I handle this situation better? (Pick one problem per meditation session.) Once you ask yourself this question, try NOT to think about it while you are actually meditating and see what answers just bubble up from your unconscious mind either during the meditation or afterwards.

1.

2.

3.

What answers came up for you on each problem.

1.

2.

3.

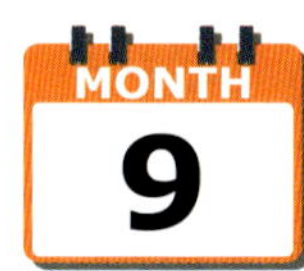

You are now meditating 20 minutes per day while adding in two extra (long) 20 to 30-minute sessions per week. Remember the issues you were having trouble with last month? Were they resolved? If so, how? Write in exactly how these problems were resolved in the lines below. If they were not resolved, reread Chapter 4 for at least three techniques that might help you cope better with your most troubling issue over the coming month.

1.

2.

3.

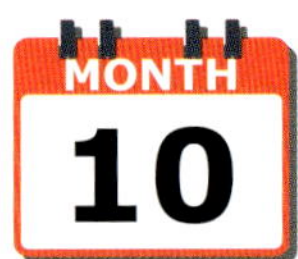

Are you ready to have one 20- minute meditation session per day, plus your other two 5-minute sessions? If so, add it into your schedule and there's no need to have the extra 20 to 30 minutes sessions twice a week since you'll already be doing that every day. Reread Chapter 9 on dealing with addictions. Think of a simple habit loop you'd like to break, whether that's snacking in between meals, or reducing the time spent on social media. Think of anything that might cue your unwanted behavior pattern, and then think what mindful steps you can take to interrupt the undesired habit loop.

Habit loop you'd like to break

Cues that trigger the habit loop

Mindfulness strategies that might help you interrupt the loop

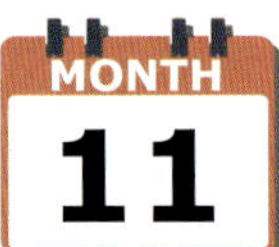

If you weren't ready to start meditating for at least 20 minutes in one session per day last month, add that in this month. So now you are meditating for one 20-minute session plus two 5-minute sessions for a total of 30 minutes a day. Or you can combine the two 5-minute sessions into one 10-minute session if you prefer, so you are meditating only twice a day rather than three. The goal, of course is to do what works best for you. If you think it would work best to simply meditate once a day, you can do that too. The point is, now you are ready to make this YOUR OWN practice.

If this is a schedule you can stick with on most days, you will start to experience some of the trait changes I wrote about in Chapter 3, if you can keep this regular meditation practice in place. If you'd like, add in one RETREAT day per month. Reread parts of Chapter 13 to see what I did on my retreat with Jon Kabat-Zinn, particularly during the silent part. Maybe you'd like to have a technology-free day, for example. Maybe you'd like to try meditating for a whole hour, do yoga for an hour and then come back and meditate more. Maybe you'd like to try eating healthy for one whole day or exercise twice in one day and take a long shower or hot bath in between. This retreat day is yours to create in any way you'd like. Pick a day, where you can be free of ALL responsibilities (like going to the store, taking care of kids, doing household chores) for at least 8 hours.

Retreat Date

Choose a day that is at least a week away from now and mark it in your calendar. **My retreat day is going to be on:**

Some of the things I'd like to do on that day include:

MONTH 12

You have been meditating for almost a whole year now! List three changes in your behavior and/or your level of inner peace and happiness that you have noticed about yourself over the last 11 months. Don't forget to mention the increase in willpower required to get you to this point.

1.

2.

3.

Now list three things from this book that helped you get to where you are today:

1.

2.

3.

Now think of three things you'd like to work on over the next twelve months:

1.

2.

3.

Find three more strategies from the book that will help you get there:

1.

2.

3.

Congratulations!

You have now been meditating for a full 12 months. Chances are your meditation practice doesn't require NEARLY as much willpower to keep in place as it did 12 months ago. In fact, you may have gotten to the point where you are experiencing many of the benefits of meditation first-hand, and as a result, you're probably not in ANY danger of slipping back into your old routines. **That's the power of a daily habit.**

Remember the quote from Aristotle in the first chapter:

First you make your habits and then your habits make you.

You are now well on your way to a thorough remodeling of your own nervous system, having already laid down new neural pathways that will enhance your sense of wellbeing, your willpower, your peace of mind, and your general levels of happiness. Over time, with continued practice, these feelings will only grow stronger and stronger.

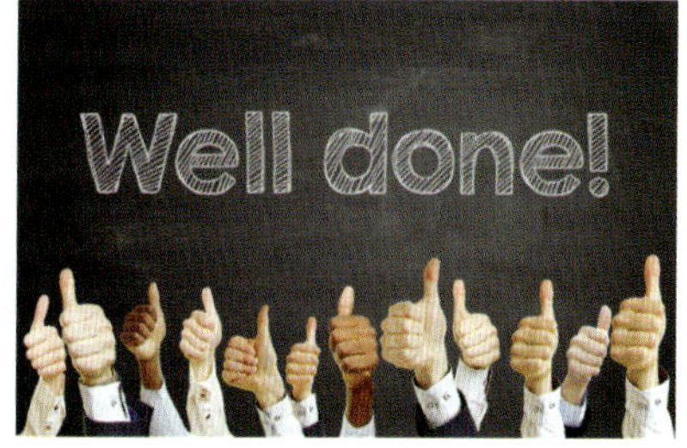

Endnotes

Chapter 1

1-1 Effects of stress on the body: "Chronic Stress Puts Your Health at Risk," Mayo Clinic Staff (see www.MayoClinic.org)

1-2 Why rumination is linked to depression: "Different Effects of Rumination on Depression: Key Role of Hope," Haitao Sun, Ph.D., et al, International Journal of Mental Health Systems.

1-3 Benefits of mindfulness: "Altered Traits," Drs. Daniel Goleman & Richard Davidson, p. 273.

1-4 The Central Park Jogger: "The Power of the Human Heart," Trisha Meili and Dr. Jon Kabat-Zinn, Advances, Vol 20, No. 1

1-5 Awareness doesn't get angry or depressed: It turns out I got this quote all wrong as I explain in the last chapter of this book: Jon Kabat-Zinn was probably quoting Sam Harris who wrote "That which is aware of fear is not fearful; That which is aware of anger is not angry."

1-6 Treatment-Resistant depression is fastest-growing mental health problems: "Treatment Resistant Depression: A Multi-Scale, Systems Biology Approach," Dr. Bruce McEwen, et al, Neuroscience & Behavioral Reviews, Elsevier Vol. 84 pp. 272-288.

1-7 Benefits of Mindfulness: "What are the Benefits of Mindfulness?" Daphne M. Davis, Ph.D. and Jeffrey A. Hayes, Ph.D., (see www.APA.org)

Chapter 2

2-1 Mindfulness changes the structure of your brain: "Altered Traits," Drs. Daniel Goleman & Richard Davidson, p. 273.

2-2 BJ Fogg, tiny habits requires no motivation: "Forget Big Change, Start with a Tiny Habit," Dr. BJ Fogg at TedX Fremont, YouTube.

2-3 BJ Fogg linking new habit with old established habit: "Forget Big Change, Start with a Tiny Habit," Dr. BJ Fogg at TedX Fremont, YouTube.

Chapter 3

3-1 Ron Siegel trait effects vs. state effects: "The Mindfulness Solution," Dr. Ron Siegel, pp. 34-35.

3-2 Sara Lazar says you benefit from meditation even if you believe "you're no good at it." I interviewed Dr. Lazar and she told me this directly. Check out her Harvard website for more information on her work. (see: Scholar.Harvard.edu/sara_lazar)

3-3 Meditation and gene expression: "Epigenetics and the Influence of our Genes," Courtney Griffin, Ph.D., TEDx OU, YouTube.

3-4 Changes in structural function of the brain: "The Mindfulness Solution," Dr. Ron Siegel, p. 35.

3-5 10,000 new neurons every day (neurogenesis occurs until the day we die): "The Brain that Changes Itself," Norman Doidge, M.D., pp. 250-253.

3-6 Plasticity can go both ways: "The Brain that Changes Itself," Norman Doidge, M.D., p. 298.

3-7 Elissa Epel, Ph.D., talks about how chronic stress wreaks havoc in the brain: "How Chronic Stress Harms our DNA," Stacy Lu, The American Psychological Association, Vol. 45 No. 9.

3-8 Mathieu Ricard's brain was different: "Training the Brain: Cultivating Emotional Intelligence," Drs. Daniel Goleman and Richard Davidson, More than Sound Productions.

3-9 Meditating 90 seconds on and off: "Training the Brain: Cultivating Emotional Intelligence," Drs. Daniel Goleman and Richard Davidson, More than Sound Productions.

3-10 Difference in size of the left side of the PFC between meditators and non-meditators: "Training the Brain: Cultivating Emotional Intelligence," Drs. Daniel Goleman and Richard Davidson, More than Sound Productions.

3-11 Tibetan monks have unusual powers of self-control: "Altered Traits," Drs. Daniel Goleman & Richard Davidson, p. 253.

3-12 Tibetan Monks dry wet towels on their bare backs: "Meditation Changes Temperatures," William Cromie, Harvard Gazette.

3-13 Genes turned on or off by meditation: "Epigenetics and the Influence of our Genes," Courtney Griffin, Ph.D., TEDx OU, YouTube.

3-14 Chronic inflammation can affect our genetic make-up: "Emotions, Stress and the Rate of Telomere Shortening" Elissa Epel, Ph.D., UCSF-TV.

3-15 Genes get turned on for life: "Epigenetics and the Influence of our Genes," Courtney Griffin, Ph.D., TEDx OU, YouTube.

3-16 Some trait effects start occurring right away: "Altered Traits," Drs. Daniel Goleman & Richard Davidson, pp. 250-251.

3-17 Broad-based benefits of mindfulness: "Altered Traits," Drs. Daniel Goleman & Richard Davidson, pp. 249-257.

3-18 Avoiding certain lifestyle diseases marked by chronic inflammation: "Emotions, Stress and the Rate of Telomere Shortening" Elissa Epel, Ph.D., UCSF-TV.

Chapter 4

4-1 John Lennon toppermost of poppermost: (see: https://www.youtube.com/watch?v=GzzeaU6p4wI)
4-2 I me mine recorded without Paul McCartney: (see: I Me Mine, Wikipedia)

Chapter 5

5-1 NY Times article about Mark Bertolini: "At Aetna, Management by Mantra," New York Times.

5-2 Another study done at Aetna: "Effective and viable mind-body stress reduction in the workplace: A randomized controlled trial," Dr. Ruth Wolever, et al, The Journal of Occupational Medicine.

5-3 Janice Marturano story at General Mills: "Janice Marturano: Huffington Post Pioneers," Huffington Post YouTube video.

5-4 Mindfulness makes you more productive at work: "Why Mindfulness is your Greatest Productivity Tool," Larry Alton, Inc. Magazine.

5-5 You're grasping onto an old story: "Meditating about Now: On a Mindfulness Retreat with Jon Kabat-Zinn," James Porter, (see: StressStop.com/Blogs)

Chapter 6

6-1 Dr. Benson worrying about losing his job: "The Relaxation Response; Foreword to the 25th Anniversary Edition," Herbert Benson, M.D., pp. 1-2.

6-2 Benefits of TM Meditation and other relaxation techniques: "The Relaxation Response," Herbert Benson, M.D., p. 9.

6-3 Famous people who practice TM: "The New Mindfulness: Meditating with the Stars," Brooke Hauser, Time Special Edition. (See also: www.TM.org)

6-4 Harvard students can't count to ten: "A Once (and future) Meditator Tries the Relaxation Response for Stress," Lloyd Resnick, Harvard Health Publishing.

6-5 Benson's four prerequisites for meditation: "The Relaxation Response," Herbert Benson, M.D., pp. 130-131.

6-6 Dr. Green practically invented biofeedback: Neurofeedback: The First Fifty Years: Contributions of Elmer and Alyce Green to Neurofeedback and the Science of Human Consciousness, Peter A. Parks, et al, Elsevier.

6-7 Swami Rama could stop his heart: "Beyond Biofeedback," Dr. Elmer Green and Alyce Green, pp. 197-218. As it turns out Swami Rama didn't completely stop the heart, but he did stop his heart from pumping blood by putting it into a state of "atrial flutter."

6-8 Swami Rama could change the temperature on his hand in two different places: "Beyond Biofeedback," Dr. Elmer Green and Alyce Green, pp. 197-218.

6-9 Swami Rama quote about what he felt about different brain wave states: "Beyond Biofeedback," Dr. Elmer Green and Alyce Green, pp. 197-218.

6-10 What the swami remembered while asleep: "Beyond Biofeedback," Dr. Elmer Green and Alyce Green.

6-11 Diseases and disorders caused by stress: "Why Zebras Don't Get Ulcers, Robert Sapolsky, Ph.D., pp. 11-13.

Chapter 7

7-1 Autoimmune disorders flare up during times of stress: "Why Zebras Don't Get Ulcers, Robert Sapolsky, Ph.D., pp. 154-160.

7-2 50% of all insomnia is caused by stress: "Why Zebras Don't Get Ulcers, Robert Sapolsky, Ph.D., pp. 226-238.

7-3 RX.com list of side effects for Halcion, aka Triazolam: (See RX.com or MayoClinic.org for an impressive list of side effects. The Mayo clinic reports: This medicine may cause you to do things while you are still asleep that you may not remember the next morning. It is possible you could drive a car, sleepwalk, have sex, make phone calls, or prepare and eat food while you are asleep or not fully awake.)

7-4 30 minutes extra sleep a night from a sleeping pill: "Sleeping Pills for Insomnia: They May not be the Best Treatment Option," (see ChoosingWisely.org, An initiative of the American Board of Internal Medicine.)

7-5 Psoriasis and mindfulness study: "Influence of a Mindfulness Meditation-Based Stress Reduction Intervention on Rates of Skin Clearing in Patients with Moderate to Severe Psoriasis Undergoing Photo Therapy (UVB) and Photochemotherapy (PUVA)," Jon Kabat-Zinn, Ph.D., et al, Journal of Psychosomatic Medicine.

7-6 Cognitive Behavioral Therapy as effective as SSRIs: "Cognitive behavioral therapy can be as effective as second-generation antidepressants to treat major depressive disorder," Science Daily.

7-7 Anti-depressants no better than a placebo in treating mild to moderate depression: Antidepressant Drug Effects and Depression Severity: A Patient-Level Meta-analysis, Steven D. Hollon, PhD; et al, JAMA Network.

7-8 Placebo meniscus surgery: "Arthroscopic partial meniscectomy versus placebo surgery for a degenerative meniscus tear: a 2-year follow-up of the randomized controlled trial," Raine Sihvonen, Ph.D., et al, Annals of the Rheumatic Diseases.

7-9 When your doctor tells you it's a placebo it can still work: "Placebo effect works, even when you know you've been given a dummy pill," Sarah Knapton, Science Editor, The Telegraph.

7-10 A. Schweitzer quote: "Each patient carries their own doctor inside of him. We are at our best when we allow this doctor to do its work." (see. Books.google.com)

7-11 medical benefits of MBSR: "What are the Benefits of Mindfulness?" Daphne M. Davis, PhD, and Jeffrey A. Hayes, PhD, (see www.APA.org)

Chapter 8

8-1 Each bout makes you more likely to have another bout: "Treatment Resistant Depression: A Multi-Scale, Systems Biology Approach," Dr. Bruce McEwen, et al, Neuroscience & Behavioral Reviews, Elsevier Vol. 84 pp. 272-288.

8-2 McEwen 50% of depression is treatment resistant: "Treatment Resistant Depression: A Multi-Scale, Systems Biology Approach," Dr. Bruce McEwen, et al, Neuroscience & Behavioral Reviews, Elsevier Vol. 84 pp. 272-288.

8-3 Getting well is only half the problem. Staying well is the other half: "The Mindful Way Through Depression," Zindel Segal, TEDx Talk.

8-4 Marsha Linehan, DBT and success rate: "The effectiveness of 6 versus 12-months of dialectical behavior therapy for borderline personality disorder: the feasibility of a shorter treatment and evaluating responses (FASTER) trial protocol," Shelley F. McMain, Ph.D., BMC Psychiatry.

8-5 Thoughts and emotions make person spiral down: "The Mindful Way Through Depression," Zindel Segal, TEDx Talk.

8-6 Albert Ellis when you realize you have an irrational thought all you have to do is change it: "How to Keep People From Pushing Your Buttons." Albert Ellis, Ph.D., p. 27.

8-7 Sadness is an incubator for depression: "The Mindful Way Through Depression," Zindel Segal, TEDx Talk.

8-8 Mindfulness is the perfect solution: Mindfulness-Based Cognitive Therapy for Depression, Second Edition.

8-9 Amygdala bigger or smaller depending on meditation: Stress reduction correlates with structural changes in the amygdala, James Carmody, Ph.D., et al, Journal of Social Cognitive and Affective Neuroscience.

Chapter 9

9-1 Judson Brewer's definition of addiction: "Everyday Addictions," Judson Brewer, M.D., Ph.D., YouTube.

9-2 Hacking the cycle of craving and addiction: "A Simple Way to Break a Bad Habit," Judson Brewer, M.D., Ph.D., TEDMED.

9-3 Getting a smoker to want to quit: "A Simple Way to Break a Bad Habit," Judson Brewer, M.D., Ph.D., TEDMED.

9-4 Dopamine as a reinforcer: "Role of brain dopamine in food reward and reinforcement," Roy A Wise, Ph.D., The Royal Society Publishing.

9-5 Habit loop can be pleasant or unpleasant: "Everyday Addictions," Judson Brewer, M.D., Ph.D., YouTube.

9-6 Looking for cues to break a habit loop: "The Power of Habit," Charles Duhigg, p. 275-286.

9-7 Coping with stress-related disease is stressful: "Disease-Proof," David Katz, M.D., MPH, p. 216-218

9-8 What Michelle Segar says about exercising and lowering stress: "Sustainable Change," Michelle Segar, (see video: MichelleSegar.com/wp/organizations)

9-9 Things that require willpower give you willpower: "The Willpower Instinct," Kelly McGonigle, Talks at Google.

9-10 RAIN acronym: "Craving to Quit," Interview with Judson Brewer, M.D., Ph.D., Mindful.org.

Chapter 10

10-1 Jon Kabat-Zinn sitting perfectly still and in pain: "Altered Traits," Drs. Daniel Goleman & Richard Davidson, p. 83.

10-2 The pain dissolved into pure sensations: "Altered Traits," Drs. Daniel Goleman & Richard Davidson, p. 84.

10-3 The pain on off switch for low level pain of itching: "Why Zebras Don't Get Ulcers, Robert Sapolsky, Ph.D., pp. 189-191.

10-4 Elissa Epel talking about how pain fluctuates: "How Chronic Stress Harms our DNA," Stacy Lu, The American Psychological Association, Vol. 45 No. 9.

10-5 Phantom limb pain: "The Tell-Tale Brain," V.S. Ramachandran, Ph.D., p. 35.

10-6 Phantom limb pain through minimizing lens: "The Tell-Tale Brain," V.S. Ramachandran, Ph.D., p. 36.

10-7 Learning how to live with pain: "Full Catastrophe Living," Jon Kabat-Zinn, Ph.D., p. 286.

10-8 Studies of pain patients at UMASS clinic: "Full Catastrophe Living," Jon Kabat-Zinn, Ph.D., pp. 288-291.

10-9 MBSR group experienced major improvements: "Full Catastrophe Living," Jon Kabat-Zinn, Ph.D., pp. 288-291.

Chapter 11

No footnotes.

Chapter 12

12-1 People who went to visit or were influenced by Neem Karoli Baba: (see: https://en.wikipedia.org/wiki/Neem_Karoli_Baba, Notable Disciples) Interestingly, Dan Goleman's name is not mentioned on this Wikipedia page. Dan told me that he had met Neem Karoli Baba on several occasions while he was in India traveling with Ram Dass.

12-2 List of qualities of self-actualizers: (See: https://en.wikipedia.org/wiki/Self-actualization.)

12-3 Seeing what we already believe: "Seeing What You Believe, Believing What You See," Deepak Chopra, Forbes.
12-4 Native Americans seeing ships as floating islands: "Native Americans first view whites from shore." Colin Calloway, American Heritage (See: https://www.americanheritage.com/native-americans-first-view-whites-shore)

12-5 Dramatically lifts the upper limits of human possibility: "Altered Traits," Drs. Daniel Goleman & Richard Davidson, p. 8.

12-6 Paul Ekman conversation with Dan Goleman about M. Ricard debate: "Knowing our Emotions, Improving Our World," Drs. Daniel Goleman and Paul Ekman, More than Sound Productions.

12-7 Eckhart Tolle on getting to enlightenment: "The New Earth," Eckhart Tolle, pp. 279-309.

Chapter 13

13-1 On retreat with Jon Kabat-Zinn: "On a Mindfulness Retreat with Jon Kabat-Zinn," James Porter, StressStop.com. I went on a six-day retreat with Jon Kabat Zinn and 35 other people. I took copious notes during the talks he would give before each meditation session. Any remarks he made that appear in quotes were jotted down by me, while he spoke, and are as accurate as I could make them. I was not recording the sessions, so it's possible that I may have made some minor errors, as I pointed out in Chapter 14.

Chapter 14

14-1 The better you get at meditating the easier it is to do: "Altered Traits," Drs. Daniel Goleman & Richard Davidson, p. 283.

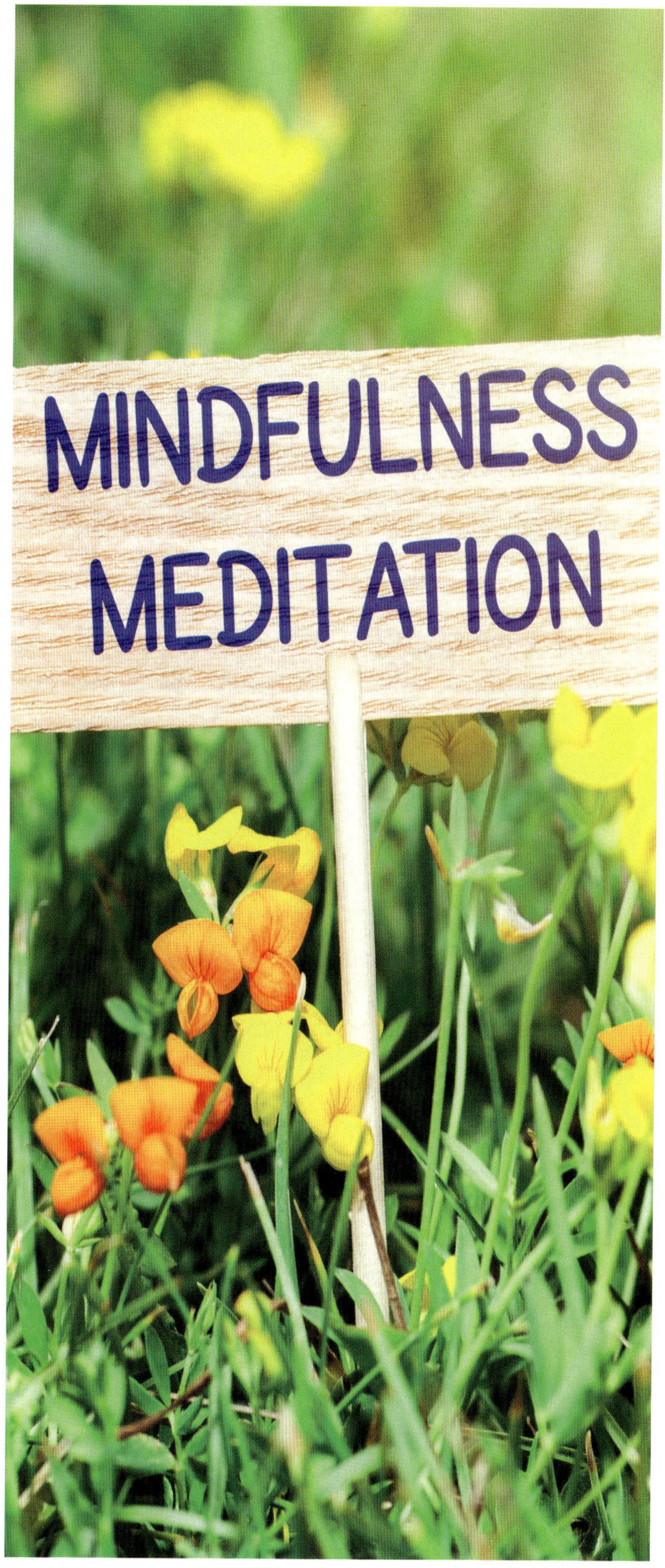

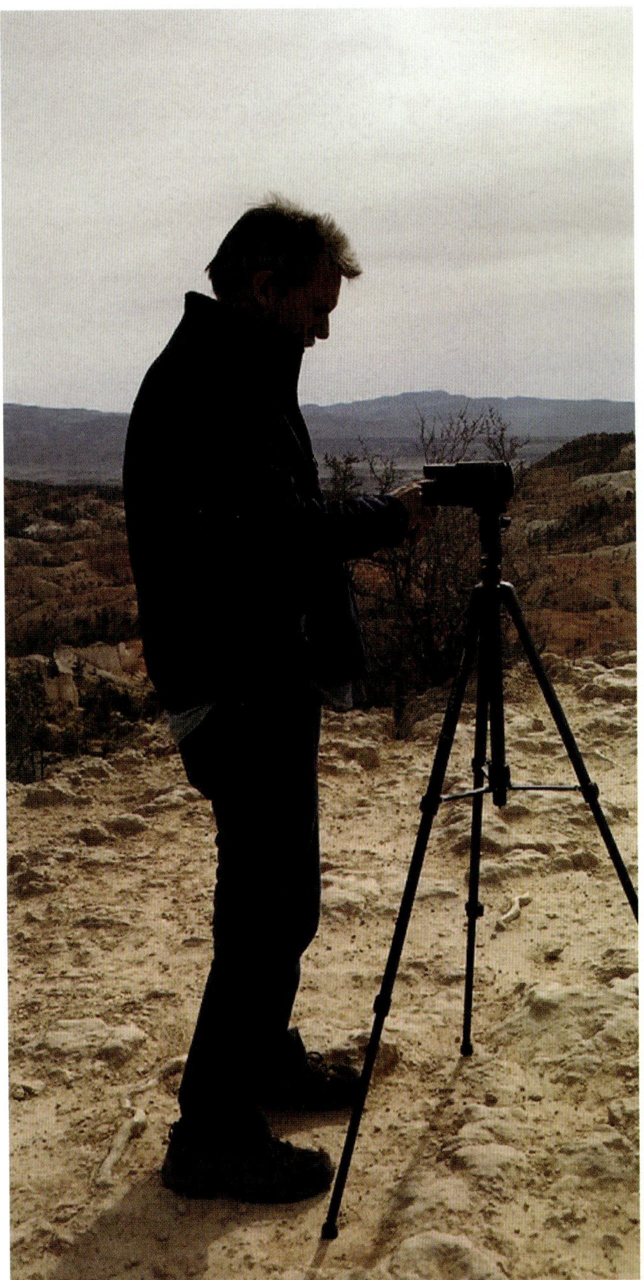

James Porter, CEO of StressStop at Bryce Canyon, Utah

If you would like to know more about the StressStop product line please go to the website: ***StressStop.com***

If you have questions for Mr. Porter or would like to have him as a speaker (or as a webinar presenter) for your organization, please contact him at: ***Jim@StressStop.com***

About The Company StressStop

James Porter founded his company, StressStop, in 1989. Working previously for another company, he created the very first relaxation video back in 1984. By the early 1990's he had created three best-selling relaxation videos and one training video which he sold to hospitals and health care facilities. Collectively, his videos have been purchased by over 3000 hospitals nationwide.

StressStop soon started offering other stress management tools and relaxation resources to an ever-expanding list of customers. These products include biodots, stress testing cards, a stress assessment called **The Stress Profiler**, a relaxation audio called **A Day Away from Stress** and a whole line of training videos on stress management, emotional intelligence and mindfulness.

That focus on educational content eventually led to the creation of a stress management web platform called **MY STRESS TOOLS** that is currently being used by corporations, hospitals, government agencies and military bases throughout the United States. And, as of the publication of this book, it's now being offered by subscription to individuals as well.